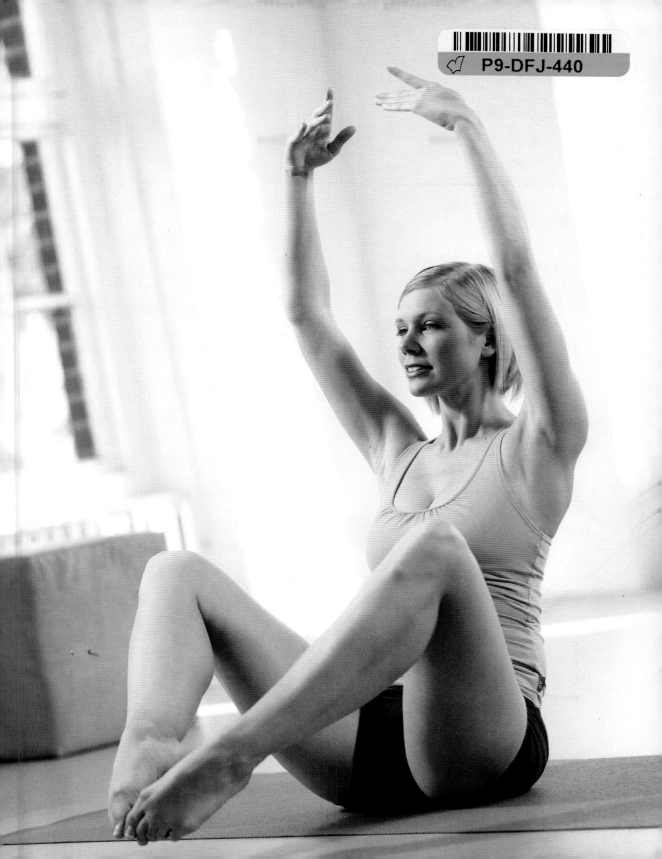

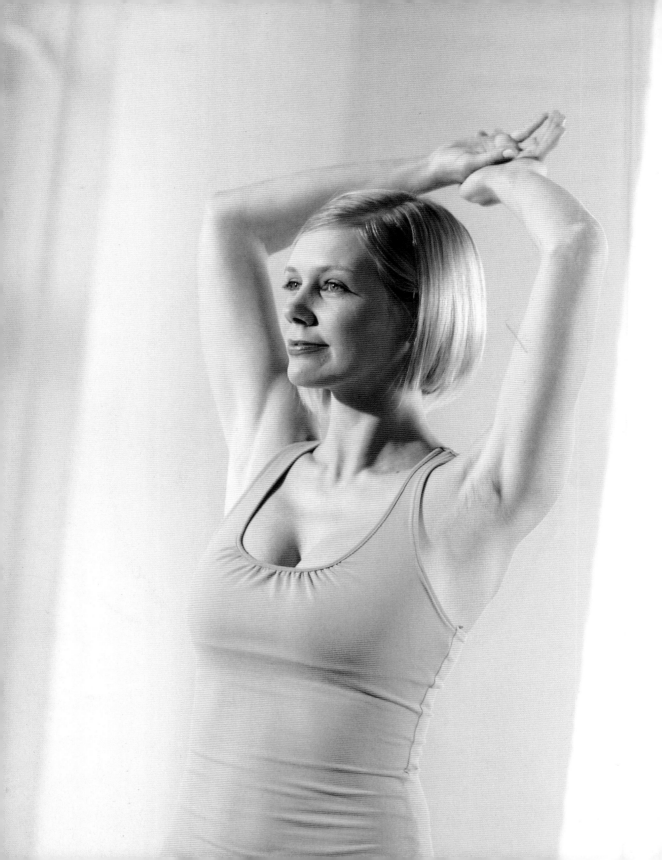

15 minute
home
Workout

Everyday Pilates
by Alycea Ungaro

Abs Workout
by Joan Pagano

Better Back Workout
by Suzanne Martin

Total Body Workout
by Joan Pagano

Gentle Yoga
by Louise Grime

DK

London, New York, Melbourne, Munich and Delhi

Senior Editor Jennifer Latham
Senior Art Editor Susan Downing
Editorial Assistant Erin Boeck Motum
Managing Editor Dawn Henderson
Managing Art Editor Christine Keilty
Art Director Peter Luff
Publisher Mary-Clare Jerram

Stills Photography Ruth Jenkinson
DTP Designer Sonia Charbonnier
Senior Production Controller Alice Holloway
Senior Production Editor Jennifer Murray
Senior Jacket Creative Nicola Powling
US Editor Rebecca Warren

DVD produced for Dorling Kindersley by
Chrome Productions www.chromeproductions.com

First American edition, 2010

Published in the United States by
DK Publishing, 375 Hudson Street
New York, New York 10014

11 12 10 9 8 7 6 5 4

009—176049—January 2010

Health warning
All participants in fitness activities must assume the
responsibility for their own actions and safety. If you have
any health problems or medical conditions, consult with
your physician before undertaking any of the activities set
out in this book. The information contained in this book
cannot replace sound judgement and good decision
making, which can help reduce risk of injury.

Published in Great Britain by
Dorling Kindersley Limited

A catalog record for this book is
available from the Library of Congress

ISBN 978-0-7566-5734-5

DK books are available at special
discounts when purchased in
bulk for sales promotions,
premiums, fundraising, or
educational use. For details,
contact: DK Publishing Special
Markets, 375 Hudson Street,
New York, New York 10014
or SpecialSales@dk.com

Printed and bound in China
by Leo Paper Group

Discover more at
www.dk.com

contents

>> **how to** use this book

The 20 programs in this book have each been specially designed to give you a well-rounded workout in 15 minutes. With step-by-step photographs and clear instructions for each exercise, these routines are the closest you can get to having a personal trainer right by your side.

In each of the 15-minute programs, the photographs capture the essence of the exercises in simple step-by-step images. Some exercises require two or three images, while others only need one. Certain exercises contain smaller inset photos that depict the first step, or starting position; in Gentle Yoga (pp306–374), they may also show a

transitional pose, the next stage of a pose, or a pose from a different angle. This is to make the sequence clearer for you to follow. You will also find targeted "feel-it-here" graphics (marked by white dotted lines) on specific exercises. These are intended to emphasize the fact that there is always a different area of the body to focus on.

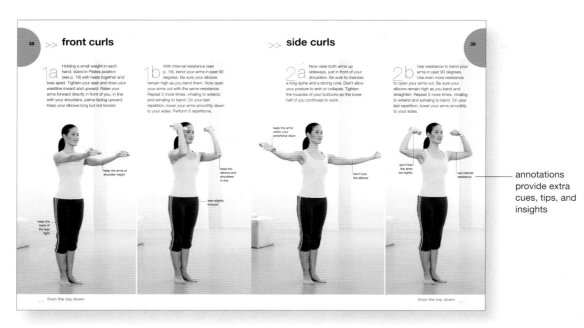

annotations provide extra cues, tips, and insights

The step-by-steps These work from left to right as you follow the step-by-step exercises. Be certain you understand the beginning and end positions before progressing.

The at-a-glance charts

The at-a-glance charts help you see each program in full view. Once you've practiced each move thoroughly, these charts will become invaluable. Use them as a quick reference to trim your practice down to a succinct 15 minutes.

The DVD

The accompanying DVD is designed to be used with the book to reinforce some of the programs shown there. The DVD demonstrates six of the routines featured in the book—Up, Up, and Away (pp. 66–79) from Everyday Pilates; Beach Ball (pp. 108–123) from Abs Workout; Energizing the Back (pp. 198–213) from Better Back Workout; the Toning Ball Workout (pp. 256–271) and Hop, Jig, and Jump (pp. 272–289) from Total Body Workout;

and the Strengthening sequence (pp. 334–345) from Gentle Yoga. As you watch the DVD, page references to the book flash up on the screen. Refer to these pages for more detailed instructions.

Exercising effectively

The programs in Everyday Pilates, Better Back Workout, and Gentle Yoga are suitable to practice every day if you wish to do so. The programs in Abs Workout and Total Body Workout should be performed with a rest day in between. Muscles need one full day of rest in between strength-training workouts, as the recovery time is just as important to the development of muscle as the exertion. For maximum results, you can do 30 minutes of moderate cardio exercise, such as swimming, walking, or cycling, on your "off" days.

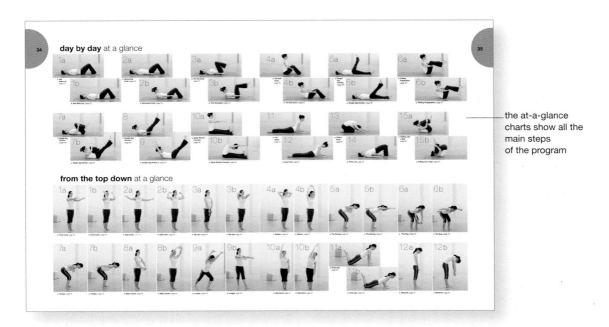

the at-a-glance charts show all the main steps of the program

At-a-glance charts These will help guide you along once you no longer need the step-by-step images. It is best to review the full program before beginning.

>> **safety** issues

Before you start any training program, you must make sure that it is safe for you to begin. First, take the PAR-Q questionnaire on the opposite page to see if you should check with your doctor before beginning. Remember, it's always wise to consult your doctor if you're suffering from an illness or any injuries.

Test your fitness

When starting a fitness program, it's useful to see how your muscular fitness measures up by counting how many repetitions you can perform or how many seconds you can hold a contraction. The three exercises shown here will assess your muscular endurance in the lower, middle, and upper body. Record your results, noting the date, and after three months of training, repeat the tests. When you reassess yourself, perform the same version of the exercise. Before attempting the exercises, warm up first by moving briskly for five minutes.

If you are just beginning to exercise, or coming back to it after a long break, you may prefer to perform your first assessment after two or three months of exercising on a regular basis.

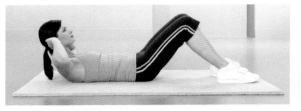

Middle body *Crunch with Scoop*
Count how many crunches you can do consecutively without resting. This is not a full sit-up. Lift your head and shoulders no higher than 30 degrees off the mat.

Your score

Excellent	50 reps or more
Good	35–49 reps
Fair	20–34 reps
Poor	20 reps or less

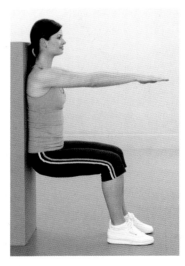

Lower body

Wall Squat
Slide down until your thighs are parallel to the floor and hold the position for as long as you can. (If you cannot slide all the way down, go as far as you can.)

Your score

Excellent	90 seconds or more
Good	60 seconds
Fair	30 seconds
Poor	less than 30 seconds

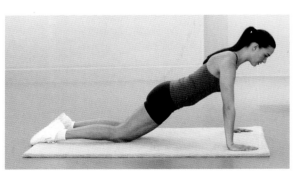

Upper body *Half Push-up*
Inhale as you bend your elbows, lowering your chest to the floor. Exhale as you push up to the starting position. Count how many you can do consecutively without a rest.

Your score

Excellent	20 reps or more
Good	15–19 reps
Fair	10–14 reps
Poor	10 reps or less

PAR-Q AND YOU A questionnaire for people aged 15 to 69 Physical Activity Readiness Questionnaire – PAR-Q (revised 2002)

Regular physical activity is fun and healthy, and increasingly more people are starting to become more active every day. Being more active is perfectly safe for most people. However, some people should check with their doctor before they start becoming much more physically active than they are already.

If you are planning to become much more physically active than you are now, start by answering the seven questions in the box below. If you are between the ages of 15 and 69, the PAR-Q will tell you if you should check with your doctor before you start. If you are over 69 years of age, and you are not used to being very active, check with your doctor.

Common sense is your best guide when you answer these questions. Please read the questions carefully and answer each one honestly: check YES or NO.

YES NO

1 Has your doctor ever said that you have a heart condition <u>and</u> that you should only do physical activity recommended by a doctor?

2 Do you feel pain in your chest when you do physical activity?

3 In the past month, have you had chest pain when you were not doing physical activity?

4 Do you lose your balance because of dizziness or do you ever lose consciousness?

YES NO

5 Do you have a bone or joint problem (for example, back, knee, or hip) that could possibly be made worse by a marked change in your physical activity?

6 Is your doctor currently prescribing drugs (for example, water pills) for your blood pressure or heart condition?

7 Do you know of any other reason why you should not do physical activity?

If you answered YES to one or more questions

Talk with your doctor by phone or in person BEFORE you start becoming much more physically active or BEFORE you have a fitness appraisal.
Tell your doctor about the PAR-Q and which questions you answered YES.
• You may be able to do any activity you want—as long as you start slowly and build up gradually. Or, you may need to restrict your activities to those which are safe for you. Talk with your doctor about the kinds of activities you wish to participate in and follow his/her advice.
• Find out which community programs are going to prove safe and helpful for you.

If you answered NO to all questions

If you answered NO honestly to all PAR-Q questions, you can be reasonably sure that you can:
• start becoming much more physically active—begin slowly and build up gradually. This is the safest and easiest way to go.
• take part in a fitness appraisal—this is an excellent way to determine your basic fitness so that you can plan the best way for you to live actively. It is also highly recommended that you have your blood pressure evaluated. If your reading is over 144/94, talk with your doctor before you start becoming much more physically active.

DELAY BECOMING MUCH MORE ACTIVE:
• if you are not feeling well because of a temporary illness such as a cold or a fever—wait until you feel better
• if you are or may be pregnant—talk to your doctor before you start becoming more active.

PLEASE NOTE:
If your health changes so that you then answer YES to any of the above questions, tell your fitness or health professional. Ask whether you should change your physical activity plan.

Source: Physical Activity Readiness Questionnaire (PAR-Q) © 2002. Reprinted by permission from the Canadian Society for Exercise Physiology. http://www.csep.ca/forms.asp

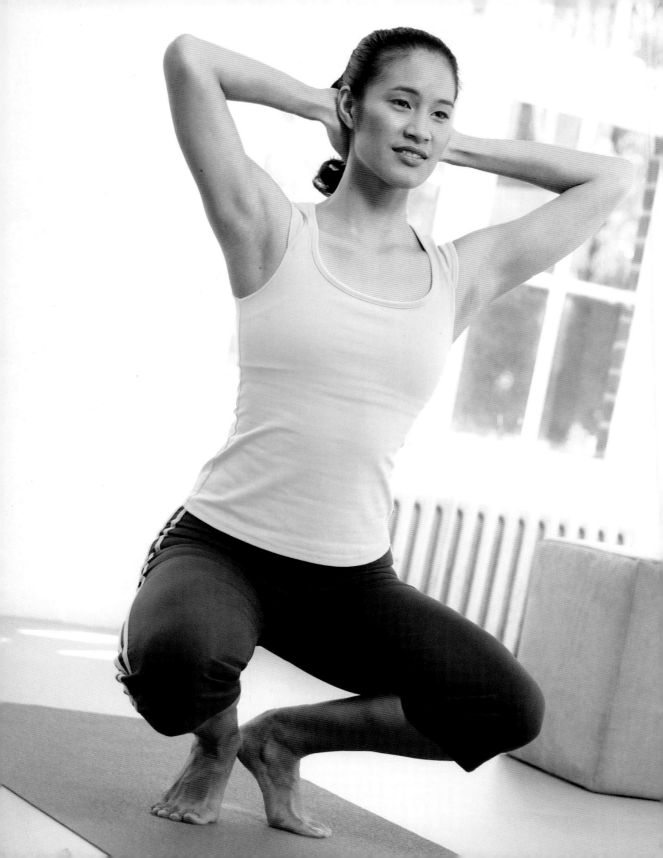

everyday
pilates

Alycea Ungaro P.T.

>> **what you need** to start

People spend so much time getting ready to exercise that many never actually do it. I have a button that reads, "I'm in no shape to exercise." This is an unfortunate and all-too common sentiment. Contrary to popular belief it is unnecessary to prepare for exercise. You simply must decide to begin.

You will need nothing more than some 2 lb (1 kg) hand weights and a well-padded mat. Since some rolling exercises can cause bruising on an unpadded surface, many yoga mats may be unsuitable. Instead, choose a mat specifically for Pilates. Finally, keep a towel handy as well as some water, and you'll be ready to go.

Clothing is next. I once had a client with knock knees who happened to be wearing pants with a seam down the front of the legs. Without thinking, I asked her to position her legs so that the seam was perfectly straight. Voilà! Her legs were better aligned and most importantly, she could see it herself. Whenever possible, select clothing with stripes or visible seams. You'll immediately notice asymmetries and will naturally correct them.

Pilates is normally performed barefoot. However, studios and health clubs often institute a footwear requirement. Bare feet are fine for the home, but for other settings, look for socks with grips to reduce slippage and protect your feet. There are even socks with compartments for each toe. Whatever you select, be sure to avoid slippery socks or cumbersome shoes that might reduce foot mobility.

Where to work out

The single largest impediment to any exercise program is inconvenience, so find yourself an area

A proper Pilates mat, a hand towel, and some small hand weights (2 lb/1 kg) are all you need to begin these Pilates programs. Be sure you have a clear space to work out in.

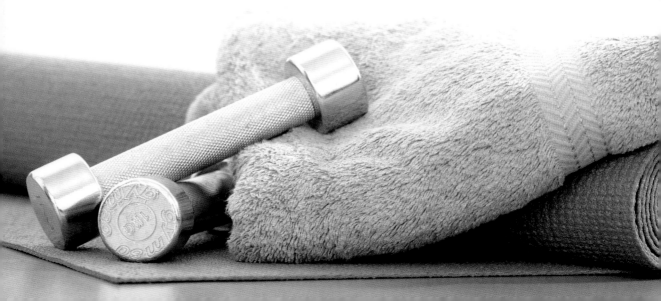

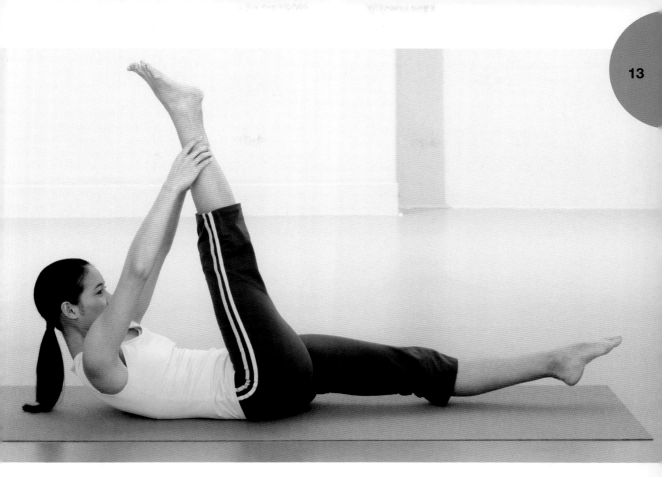

that is easy to get to and a time that is convenient for your schedule. Pilates can be done anywhere you have enough room to stretch out on a mat. You can practice at a gym or at home. You can even practice on a lawn or beach, as long as you have an appropriate mat.

The safety instinct

Have you ever heard a little voice inside your head cautioning you to stop what you were doing? Did you listen? If you did, you are probably naturally intuitive about safety. For the rest of us, developing that intuition will be largely trial and error. To keep you working out safely, here are some guidelines:

1 Begin with just one program.

2 Remember to hydrate. By the time you feel thirsty, you are already dehydrated.

3 Learn to distinguish between effort and pain. Effort is OK, pain is a signal to stop.

4 If something doesn't "feel" right, stop.

Clothing can be a visual aid as you work out. Selecting attire with stripes can help you establish good alignment and make improvements to your form.

>> **tips for** getting started

- **Don't waste time** getting ready to exercise. You are ready. Just begin.

- **If a mat is not readily available** use some folded blankets or large towels instead. Plush carpeting can also be a suitable workout surface.

- **Find a time of day** when your energy is at its lowest. Just lying down for one exercise will get your blood flowing and will give you an energy burst.

>> **pilates** from the inside out

Therapists train their patients to become self-aware. This is a significant step toward mental and emotional well-being. Similarly, exercise instructors teach you to become physically self-aware. By recognizing your habits and body mechanics, you can embark upon a path of physical health and well-being.

Your body is amazing. The coordination of events required for simple actions such as bending your knee or opening your hand is astonishing, yet they happen without us noticing a thing.

By contrast, Pilates teaches your mind to train your body very consciously. During the programs you will continually be required to recognize your positions, make adjustments and note your physical sensations. In addition, you must also be focused on the order of exercises, so that you can anticipate and prepare for the next move.

This "mind–body" connection often suggests a workout that is neither physical nor rigorous, but Pilates is both. Just because we think our way through Pilates does not make it less taxing on the muscles. In fact, just the opposite is true. In the words of the late Frederick Schiller, "It is the mind itself that builds the body." Joseph Pilates, the founder of Pilates, was quite fond of this saying.

Learning new patterns

Our brains are built to learn new patterns. As we learn new skills, connections between previously unconnected brain cells are formed. Repetition is key. Each time you do a correct abdominal curl you are building a connection that makes it easier to do correctly the next time. In sum, "cells that fire together, wire together."

Pilates trains this mind-to-body dialog. You will learn to direct your actions on a gross motor scale as well as a fine motor scale so your results will be amplified and expedited.

>> **just make it** happen

- **Pay attention to your body** throughout your day. Self-awareness is key to good health. If you watch how you move, your exercise routine will improve.

- **Exercise is an activity.** It is not something that happens to you—you make it happen.

- **It requires more energy to avoid** something than simply to do it. Don't waste any time making excuses. Just hit the mat and get started!

Your Pilates body

As you read this book and progress through the workouts, you will find instructions for and mentions of specific parts of your body. The chart opposite is a handy reference guide to them. For ease of use, we have chosen layperson terms rather than anatomical ones. Names and labels allow your mind to grasp more effectively what is required of you, so become familiar with them and use them as you move through your workout. Think of the chart as a map for your mind.

Remember these simple names for your body parts. Learning about your anatomy will help you identify trouble spots as well as areas of strength in your body.

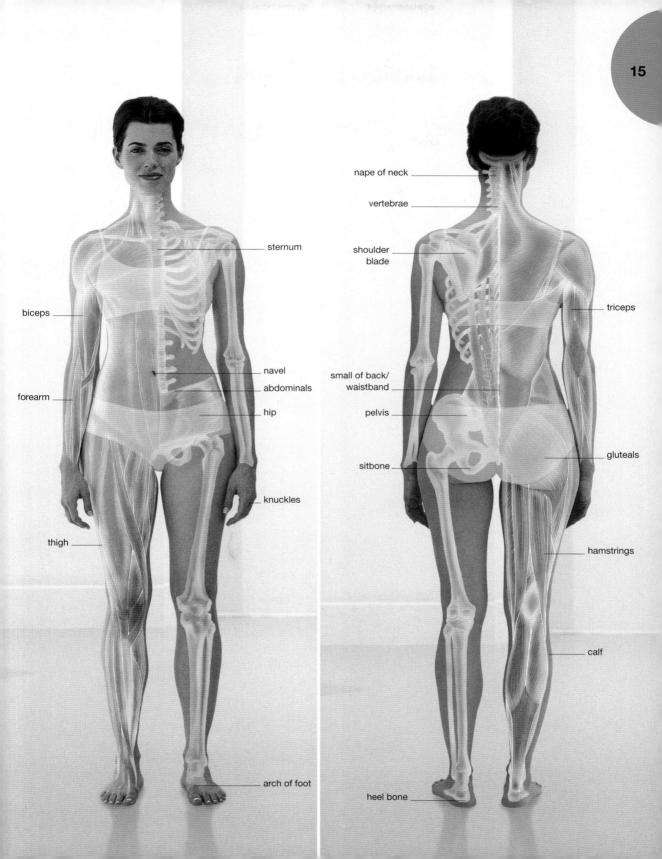

sternum

nape of neck

vertebrae

shoulder
blade

biceps

triceps

navel

abdominals

small of back/
waistband

forearm

pelvis

hip

gluteals

sitbone

knuckles

thigh

hamstrings

calf

arch of foot

heel bone

>> **pilates** concepts

Your Pilates technique and form can constantly be improved upon. Just as musicians must rehearse tirelessly, Pilates will only get better as you train. Think of it as a language. First you learn the words, then some phrases, and finally you work on your accent. Let's begin here with your first Pilates words.

Before you can start on the mechanics of Pilates, there are six fundamental principles that you should become familiar with. These principles give substance and purpose to the workouts and help you learn to integrate your workout into your life so you begin to feel healthy and strong. Remember, the benefits of Pilates are meant to extend well beyond the actual workout.

Control
This is the primary principle of the system. In his time, Joseph Pilates called his method "Contrology." His focus on controlled movement was a result of his years of blending Eastern and Western disciplines. As you work out, control your muscles, your positions, and your tempos. Your body is your tool and by exerting control over it, it will produce better and better results.

Centering
This is a somewhat vague principle to many people. The idea is that all movement begins from your center. I'm of the mind that Pilates was really drawing on the principle that you must "stabilize before you mobilize." In Pilates we brace or stabilize the core and then mobilize the limbs. Beyond that, there is an energetic component in working from your center. It's as though you were able to harness and then project out through the limbs all of the energy and activity going on in your internal organs. Centering is akin to saying you should work from the inside out.

>> **tips for** surefire success

- **Don't over-analyze the work.** Pilates is complicated but it's meant to be a moving system. Keep moving at all costs.

- **Working out is an extension of your life.** Put the same effort into it that you would into anything else.

- **Don't work out—work in!** Inner work shapes the outer body.

- **Never say die.** If an exercise is easy, you're not working hard enough.

- **Don't ask what** an exercise is good for. Mr. Pilates said, "It's good for the body."

Concentration
Concentration is key to Pilates. Without focused concentration, any exercise can only be moderately beneficial. Concentration elevates your intensity and so takes your results up to a far higher level.

Precision
This is the fourth principle and just as many of the other principles apply globally, so "precision" serves as an umbrella for this whole list. Attention to the smallest detail is what makes Pilates so effective.

Breath

Breathing is a focus of the Pilates work. Many people come to Pilates because they have heard that it is a breathing technique. You will learn step-by-step breathing in these programs but it is not their focus. As a general rule, inhale to prepare for a movement and exhale as you execute it.

Flow of movement

This is an element that comes later in the practice but can be incorporated early on. As you learn each exercise, be sure to perform it in a seamless, flowing manner. Eventually you'll work on creating one long routine.

Minimum of movement

Other ideas and concepts, such as symmetry, balance, and integration arise as instructors make their own contributions to Pilates. All of these are applicable but Mr. Pilates clearly intended his work to be succinct, so when establishing its main tenets, he chose only the key moves and critical concepts. This working list of six incorporates all the dozens of ideas and concepts at play in Pilates.

Off the floor and out the door

Now that you've learned the six principles, think about how they apply to real life. Concepts such as control, precision, or breath can be applied to your life anywhere and anytime. Your workout should be a microcosm of how you live. If you never did any of these programs, you could still embark upon a brand-new lifestyle simply by incorporating these key principles.

Working out on your own should be just as focused as working with a trainer. Learn to be your own teacher by cueing and correcting yourself constantly.

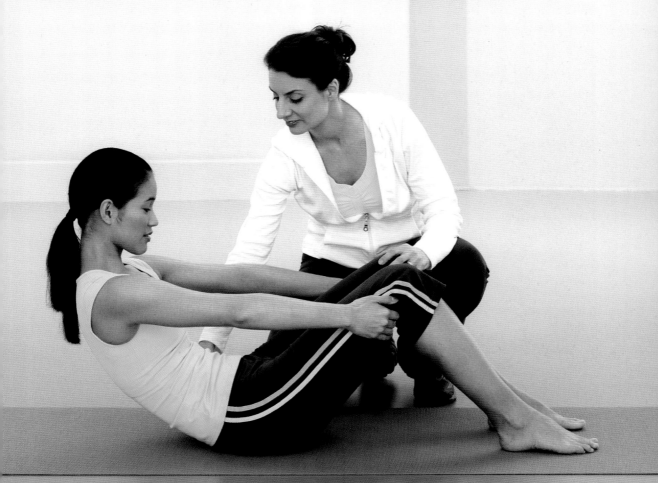

>> **pilates** top to tail

Now that we've covered the ideology of Pilates and the approach you will need to be successful, let's review the physical principles that are present throughout the programs in this series. Certain elements of positioning are specific to Pilates. Let's start at the top of the body and work our way down.

To keep your neck well aligned during abdominal work, imagine resting your head on a raised support. The curve should be long and natural both front and back. Avoid any crunching or tightening around the throat.

Your breathing in Pilates needs to be specific. The abs must work in a contracted fashion at all times so your breathing must be redirected both upward and outward. Be aware that your lungs actually extend all the way above your collarbones. Practice breathing laterally, expanding the rib cage sideways as you inhale, and then contracting it inward as you exhale.

Below the waist

Pilates teachers have several labels for the abdominals, including the core, the center, and frequently, the powerhouse. No matter the tag,

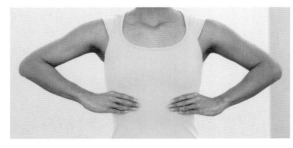

Practice breathing laterally with the hands on either side of the rib cage. On an inhale, the hands should pull apart.

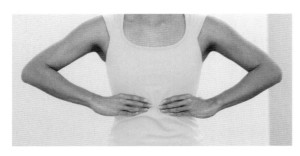

Exhale and feel the ribs narrowing. The hands draw together. Keep the abs tight.

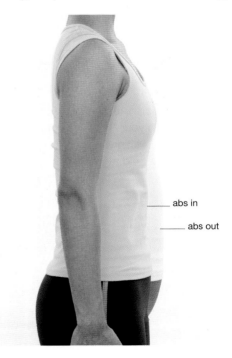

abs in

abs out

The Pilates Scoop activates the abdominal wall. Keep your waist lifted and narrowed. Never allow it to collapse.

your strength and control always spring from the center of your torso. Your powerhouse specifically incorporates your abs, hips, and buttocks as well.

The Pilates Scoop (see opposite, bottom right) is the signature of the method. Even if you have difficulty pulling the abs inward, you must never allow them to push outward.

Optimal spinal alignment means positioning your spine to preserve its natural curves. To do this, when you are lying flat for abdominal exercises, keep from tucking or curling the lower back. Instead, try to lengthen the spine. The end result should be strong, supportive abdominal muscles.

Additionally, when you are working your seat muscles or gluteals, think of "wrapping" the muscles of the buttocks and thighs around toward the back. This will create a tightening and lifting of those muscles and will help to support your spine.

Pilates position or Pilates stance doesn't happen in the feet, although it looks that way. Working from your hips down, the gluteal muscles in your rear-end and in the backs of your thighs work together to rotate and wrap around. This causes a slight opening of the toes.

Perfect the details

As you work out, focus on your symmetry. Imagine your torso in a box from shoulders to hips. If your box is square, you are likely well aligned. You also need to work within your "frame," which means keeping your limbs within your peripheral vision and never going beyond a comfortable joint range.

Never forget that Pilates is strength training. To maximize its benefits you must always work with resistance. Some resistance is provided by gravity and your positions. More important is the internal resistance you create. Your entire Pilates routine should incorporate this internal resistance.

Opposition is a final but vital ingredient of your Pilates practice. For every action there is an equal and opposite reaction. Pilates is the same. As one side reaches, another side contracts. If you lift up, you also anchor down. By using direct opposition you will find the stability and strength in your core to build a better body.

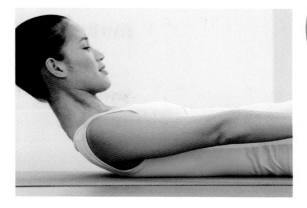

In abdominal work keep your neck lengthened and aligned. Don't force the chin down or tense the throat. Lifting the head comes from your abdominal strength.

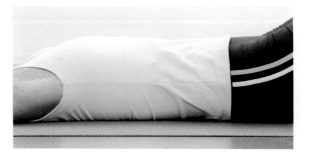

Performing exercises on your back can be tricky for your spine. When working your abs, keep your spine lengthened rather than curling it up underneath you.

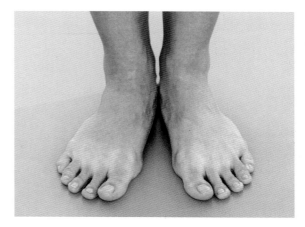

In Pilates stance the heels connect as the toes open. This is achieved by activating and rotating the buttocks muscles and the muscles in the backs of the thighs.

15 minute

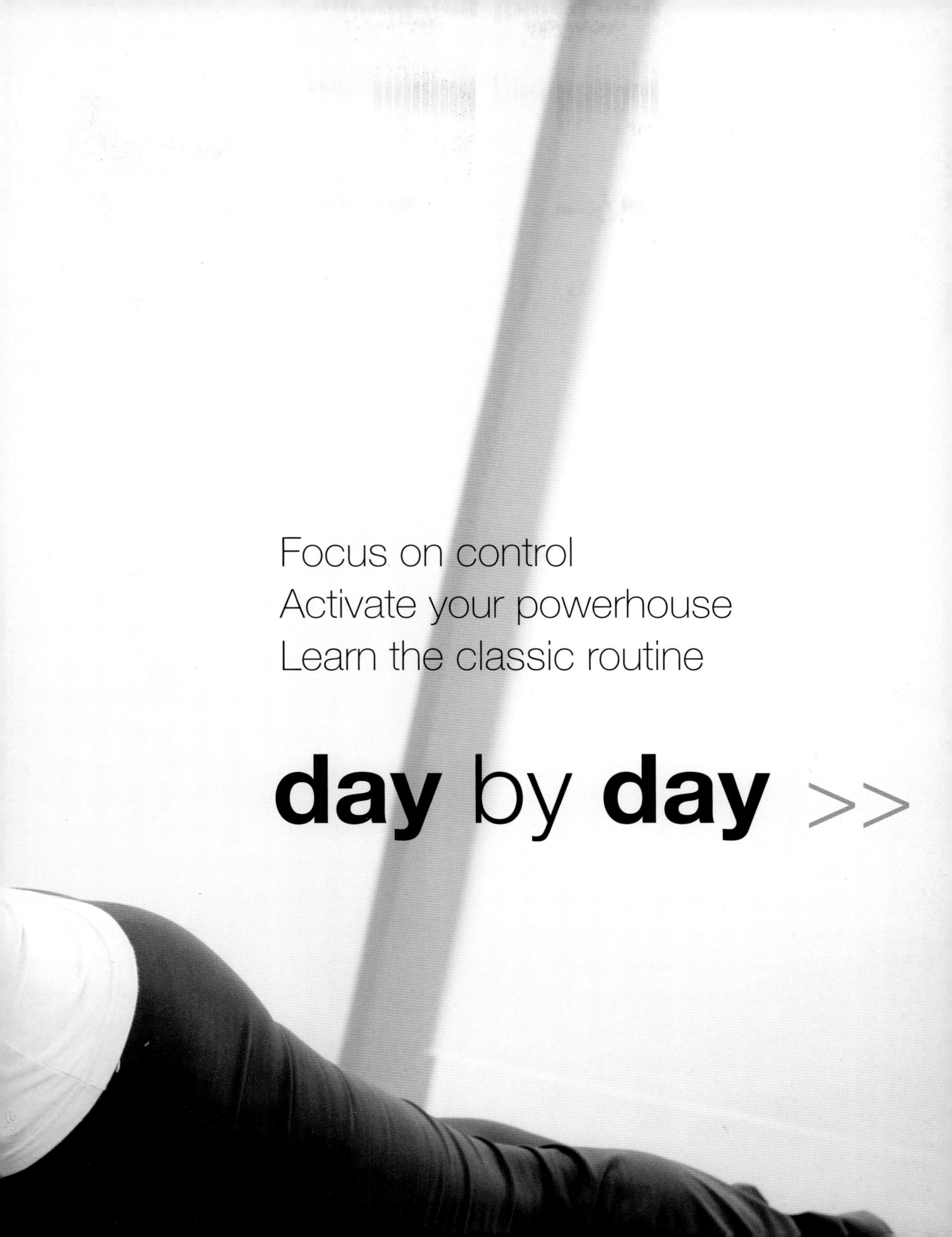

Focus on control
Activate your powerhouse
Learn the classic routine

day by **day** >>

>> **abs wake-up**

1a Lie flat with your knees bent and your hands across your abdominals. Even lying flat, your posture should be perfect. Keep your neck long, your shoulders down, and your "box" square (see p. 19). Inhale deeply and let your abs expand. Your hands will lift as you do this.

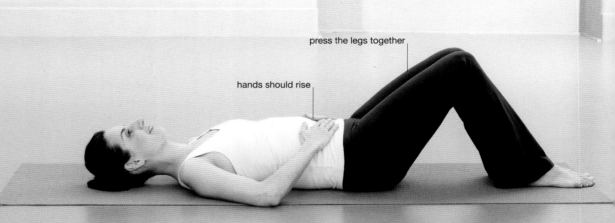

press the legs together

hands should rise

1b Now exhale completely, emptying your lungs and sinking your abs. Don't crunch your midsection or hunch your shoulders. Just pull your belly in deeper, allowing your waist to hollow out. Repeat for 4 repetitions, exhaling longer and contracting deeper with each repetition.

keep the ribs in

keep the neck long

2a Extend your arms forward so they hover just above the mat. Your feet remain firmly planted on the mat and your legs are pressed together. Your abs pull inward and upward. Prepare to curl up by inhaling.

activate
the abs

keep the arms above the mat

2b Exhale, and without letting your abdominal wall expand, lift your head, neck, and shoulders, curling up off the mat. Reach your arms longer and keep focused on your midsection. Lower down smoothly with an inhale. As you repeat, pull in your abs even further. Repeat 3 more times for a total of 4 repetitions.

keep the eyes on
the midsection

sink the abs deeper

>> **the hundred**

3a Begin with both knees drawn into your chest. Curl your upper body up off the mat and reach your arms along your sides just above the mat. Pull in your abs.

pull the abs in and up

keep the hips flat on the mat

3b Take both legs up to a 90 degree angle, with your shins parallel to the floor. Pump your arms up and down vigorously, breathing in for 5 pumps and out for 5 pumps. Continue until you reach 100, resting briefly if needed. Keep your abs deep and your torso still and strong.

point the knees straight up

keep the fingers long

>> **the roll-down**

4a Sit upright at the front of your mat, legs apart and feet flat, holding behind your thighs. Inhale and direct the back of your waistband to pull down toward the mat. Your tail will curl underneath and your abs will hollow.

draw the shoulders down ———   ——— lift the chest up

4b Keep curling your tail as you aim the small of your back to the floor. Keep your legs still. Pause at your lowest point and take 3 breaths, hollowing your abs further. Exhale and fold back up. Roll up to your tallest posture and repeat one more set.

feel it here

fold in the waist

>> single-leg circles

5a Lie flat with both your legs and arms extended. Fold your right leg in and straighten it to the sky (see inset). Fix the rest of your body solidly on the mat, stretching both knees and pressing your shoulders back and down. Cross your raised leg up and over your body, aiming for your left shoulder.

lift the leg and cross it over

press the triceps down

5b Continue making a circle with your raised leg, around and back up to center. Circle 4 more times, then reverse for another 5 repetitions. Bend your knee in, lower it, and repeat to the left side.

keep the hip of the bottom leg stable

keep the bottom leg straight

>> **rolling preparation**

6a Sit at the front edge of your mat, holding behind your thighs with your legs in the air. Keep your shins parallel to the floor. Hold your chest high and scoop your abs. Your elbows are open wide and your ankles are long.

keep the knees and feet in a line

keep the abs scooped in

6b Tip your pelvis under you, then use your abs to ease back further. At your limit, pull your abs in further and fold your waist in, rounding forward. Sit tall and repeat 3 more times. Lower your feet only after the last repetition.

curl the tail under

hollow out the midsection

>> **single-leg stretch**

7a Lie flat with both knees bent into your chest. Before you curl up, be sure your box or frame is square and then activate your powerhouse (see p. 19).

hug the knees tightly

keep the chest open

7b Curl your upper body off the mat and hold your left leg, reaching your left hand to your ankle and your other to your knee. Extend your right leg 45 degrees. Control your torso as you switch legs, inhaling on one side and exhaling on the other. Continue switching for 8 repetitions. Bend both knees to finish. Rest your head.

watch hand placement

reach the leg long

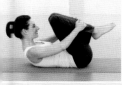

8 Curl your upper body back up and hug your ankles in tightly (see inset). Inhale to simultaneously reach your arms and legs forward. Exhale to hug them back in. Keep your upper body lifted off the mat and repeat for 4 more repetitions.

take the legs to a 45 degree angle

hold the arms at hip height

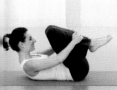

9 Repeat as before (see inset) but now add a backward reaching of your arms. Hollow your abs even deeper as you repeat the sequence. Your arms and legs now reach to a 45 degree angle. Repeat 5 times and rest.

take the arms to a 45 degree angle

tighten the abs

>> **spine stretch forward**

10a Sit tall at the front of your mat with your feet just wider than the mat. Extend both arms in front of you at shoulder height and flex your feet. Tighten your rear end and inhale so you feel as though you are rising up off the mat.

press the
shoulders down

point the
toes up

10b Exhale slowly and dive over, lowering your head and reaching forward with your arms to stretch your back. As you round, keep pulling back in your waist. Inhale to return to upright. Repeat 3 more times. After the final repetition, exaggerate your height, lengthening even taller.

dive the head
through the arms

pull back
in the waist

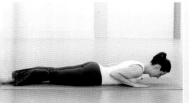

11 Lie face down with legs together and hands under your shoulders. Breathing normally, lengthen your spine forward, pressing your shoulders back away from your ears (see inset). Continue lengthening to arc up off the mat. Use your stomach muscles to support you. Lower with control. Repeat 2 more times.

legs may separate

take the elbows to a 90 degree angle

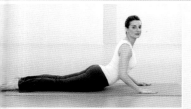

12 From your final Swan, turn your head to the right (see inset), then circle your chin down and around to the other side. Return to center looking straight ahead. Reverse. Repeat 2 more times. After 4 repetitions, lower with control.

stretch the neck

keep your weight centered

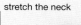

>> child's pose/pelvic lift

13 Push back to sit on your heels with your back rounded, hands in front of you. Open your knees slightly to allow your upper body to sink deeper. Keep your abs lifted as you take 3 deep breaths. With each inhale, try to stretch and release your lower-back muscles. With each exhale, draw your navel even higher upward. After 3 deep breaths, roll up to a kneeling position.

reach the hands forward

knees may open

14 Lie with knees bent and legs hip-width apart. Feel your chest open, shoulders back, and spine long (see inset). Inhale and raise your hips without arching your back. Exhale and lower down, one vertebra at a time. Repeat 3 more times, increasing the articulation of your spine each time.

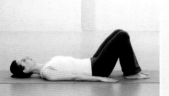

feel it here

reach the knees forward

keep the ribs in

15a

Balance on your sitbones at the front edge of your mat, hugging your ankles into your body and nestling your head between your knees (see inset). Without letting your feet touch down, tuck your tail under you and begin to roll back.

hold the ankles snugly

keep the head tucked in

15b

Keep rolling through your spine back to your shoulder blades, then return to the starting point. Use your abs for control, especially on the return. Try not to skip any sections of your spine. Repeat 5 more times, inhaling as you roll and exhaling as you return.

take the feet close to the buttocks

aim the sitbones to the sky

don't rock onto the neck

day by day at a glance

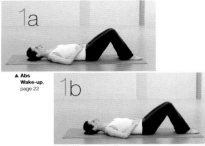

1a

▲ Abs Wake-up, page 22

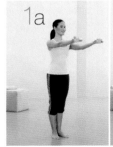

1b

▲ Abs Wake-up, page 22

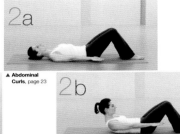

2a

▲ Abdominal Curls, page 23

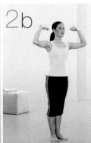

2b

▲ Abdominal Curls, page 23

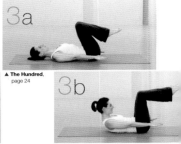

3a

▲ The Hundred, page 24

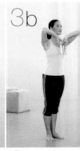

3b

▲ The Hundred, page 24

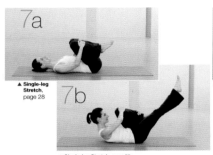

7a

▲ Single-leg Stretch, page 28

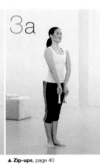

7b

▲ Single-leg Stretch, page 28

8

▲ Double-leg Stretch 1, page 29

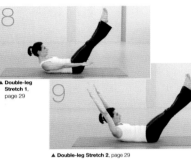

9

▲ Double-leg Stretch 2, page 29

10a

▲ Spine Stretch Forward, page 30

10b

▲ Spine Stretch Forward, page 30

from the top down at a glance

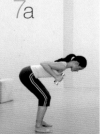

1a

▲ Front Curls, page 38

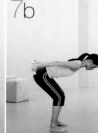

1b

▲ Front Curls, page 38

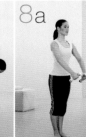

2a

▲ Side Curls, page 39

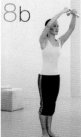

2b

▲ Side Curls, page 39

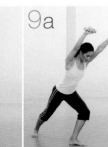

3a

▲ Zip-ups, page 40

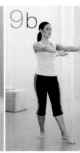

3b

▲ Zip-ups, page 40

7a

▲ Triceps, page 44

7b

▲ Triceps, page 44

8a

▲ Baby Circles, page 45

8b

▲ Baby Circles, page 45

9a

▲ Lunges, page 46

9b

▲ Lunges, page 46

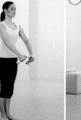

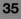

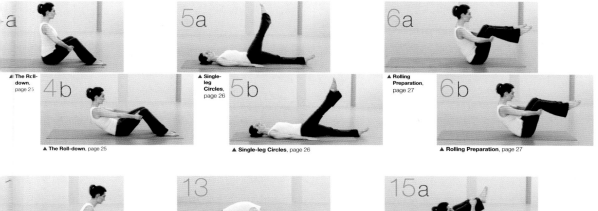

▲ The Roll-down, page 25

4b

▲ The Roll-down, page 25

5a

▲ Single-leg Circles, page 26

5b

▲ Single-leg Circles, page 26

6a

▲ Rolling Preparation, page 27

6b

▲ Rolling Preparation, page 27

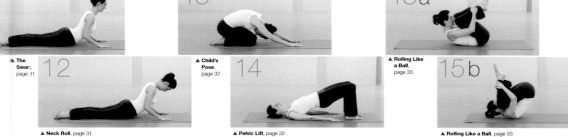

▲ The Swan, page 31

12

▲ Neck Roll, page 31

13

▲ Child's Pose, page 32

14

▲ Pelvic Lift, page 32

15a

▲ Rolling Like a Ball, page 33

15b

▲ Rolling Like a Ball, page 33

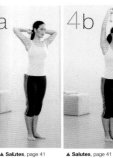

▲ Salutes, page 41

4b

▲ Salutes, page 41

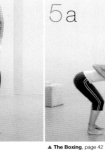

5a

▲ The Boxing, page 42

5b

▲ The Boxing, page 42

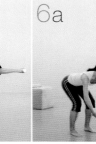

6a

▲ The Bug, page 43

6b

▲ The Bug, page 43

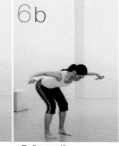

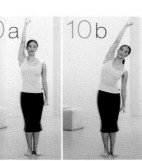

10a

▲ Side Bend, page 47

10b

▲ Side Bend, page 47

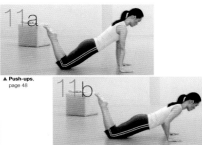

11a

▲ Push-ups, page 48

11b

▲ Push-ups, page 48

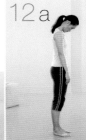

12a

▲ Windmill, page 49

12b

▲ Windmill, page 49

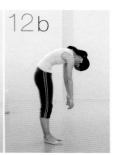

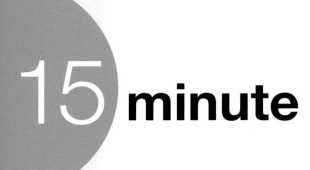

15 minute

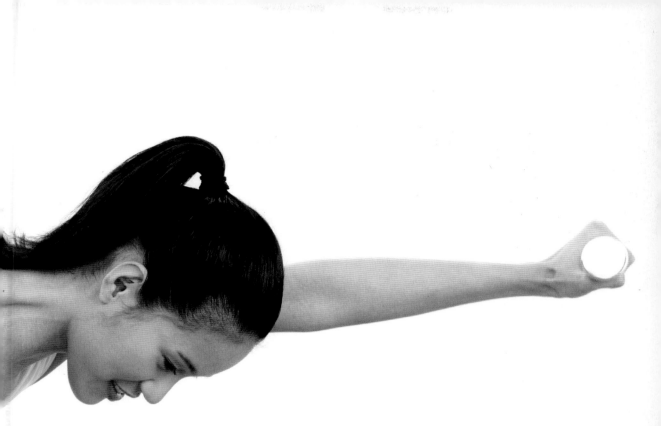

from the
top down >>

Focus on centering
Activate your Pilates box
Learn Pilates with weights

>> **front curls**

1a Holding a small weight in each hand, stand in Pilates position (see p. 19) with heels together and toes apart. Tighten your seat and draw your waistline inward and upward. Raise your arms forward directly in front of you, in line with your shoulders, palms facing upward. Keep your elbows long but not locked.

1b With internal resistance (see p. 19), bend your arms in past 90 degrees. Be sure your elbows remain high as you bend them. Now open your arms out with the same resistance. Repeat 5 more times, inhaling to extend, and exhaling to bend. On your last repetition, lower your arms smoothly down to your sides. Perform 6 repetitions.

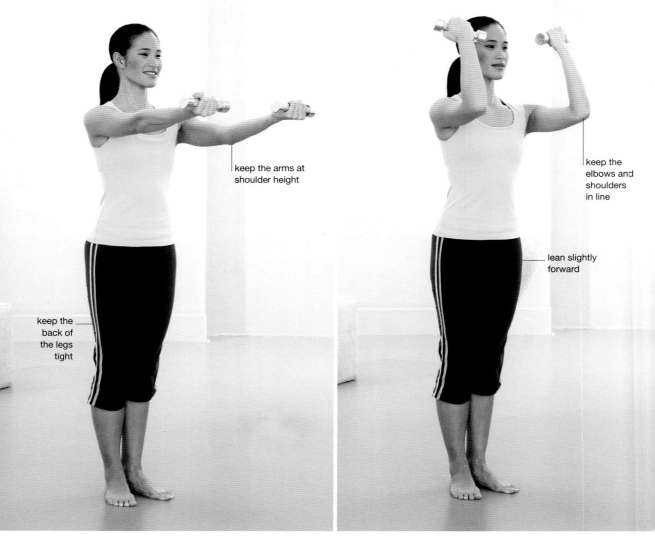

keep the arms at shoulder height

keep the elbows and shoulders in line

lean slightly forward

keep the back of the legs tight

2a Now raise both arms up sideways, just in front of your shoulders. Be sure to maintain a long spine and a strong core. Don't allow your posture to sink or collapse. Tighten the muscles of your buttocks so the lower half of you continues to work.

2b Use resistance to bend your arms in past 90 degrees. Use even more resistance to open your arms out. Be sure your elbows remain high as you bend and straighten. Repeat 5 more times, inhaling to extend and exhaling to bend. On your last repetition, lower your arms smoothly to your sides.

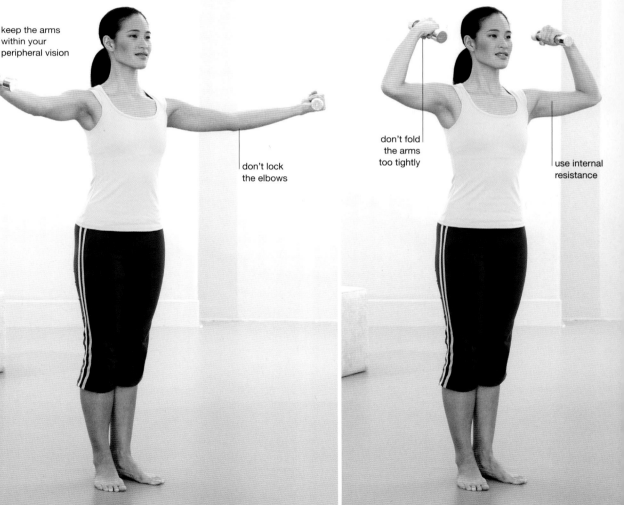

keep the arms within your peripheral vision

don't lock the elbows

don't fold the arms too tightly

use internal resistance

>> zip-ups

3a Still holding the small weights, rotate the backs of your hands toward each other so your knuckles face each other. Scoop your abs up, tighten the backs of your legs, and shift your weight a tiny bit forward toward the fronts of your feet. Keep your heels flat as you do this. Inhale to prepare.

3b Exhale, open your elbows wide, and pull the weights up under your chin, keeping your neck long and your shoulders relaxed. Lower the weights back down as though you were pushing something heavy away from you. Repeat 5 more times, inhaling to lift and exhaling to lower.

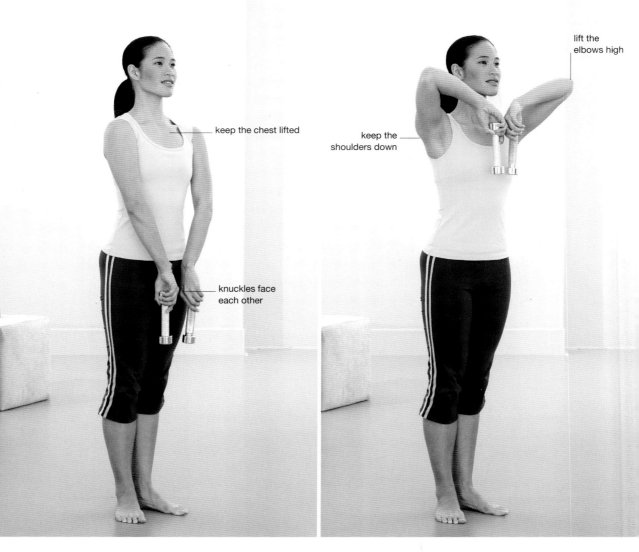

keep the chest lifted

knuckles face each other

lift the elbows high

keep the shoulders down

>> **salutes**

4a Still holding the weights, place both of them behind your head at the nape of your neck. Tip your chin down slightly and be sure to keep your elbows open wide. Your feet remain in Pilates position with your legs pressed together tightly. Incline your body forward as though you were "leaning into the wind."

4b Without locking your elbows, extend your arms overhead. Hold your powerhouse strong (see p. 19) and keep your fingers of each hand in contact with each other. Lower with resistance. Repeat 5 more times, exhaling to extend and inhaling to lower.

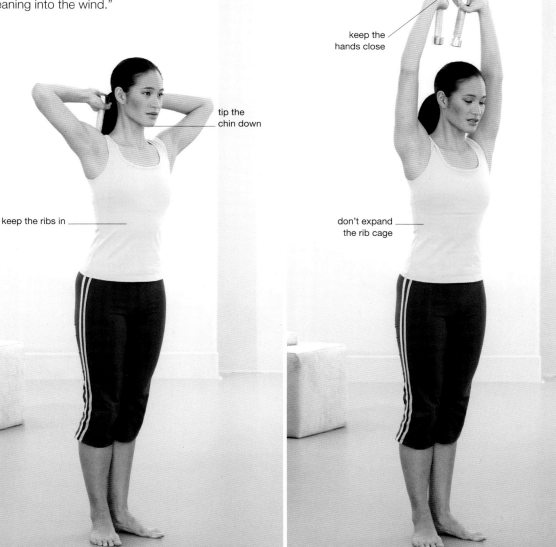

tip the
chin down

keep the ribs in

keep the
hands close

don't expand
the rib cage

>> **the boxing**

5a Open your feet into parallel, hip-width apart, and stand tall holding the weights (see inset). Bend both knees deeply and fold over your legs with a long flat back. Tuck your arms in by your sides, keeping your elbows tight to your body. Lift your abs without disrupting your posture. Inhale to prepare.

5b Exhale and simultaneously extend your right arm forward and your left arm back in a boxinglike movement. Inhale to fold your arms back in. Continue, creating resistance and alternating sides for 3 full sets. Complete a total of 6 repetitions. To finish, round over your legs, stretching your back and legs. Slowly roll back up to standing.

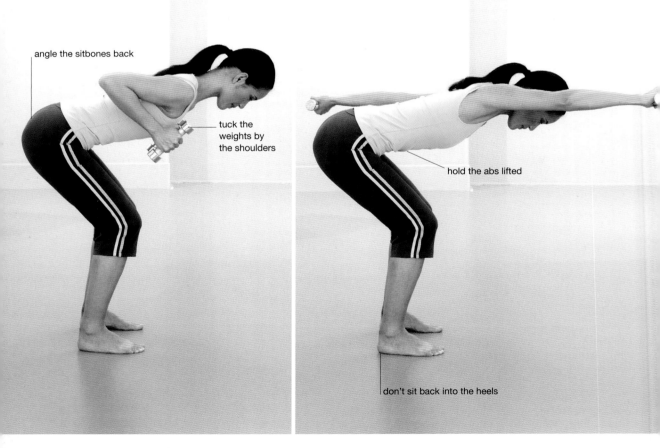

angle the sitbones back

tuck the weights by the shoulders

hold the abs lifted

don't sit back into the heels

>> **the bug**

6a Start by standing tall, holding the weights, and with legs parallel. Bend your knees and fold over, keeping your spine long and flat. Frame your arms in a circle directly underneath you, bringing your fists toward each other. Lift your powerhouse and inhale to prepare.

6b Exhale and lift both arms to the sides of the room. Don't allow your body position to change as you do this. Inhale and lower your arms as though you were squeezing something together. Perform 2 more repetitions, then reverse your breathing and exhale to prepare for an additional 3 repetitions. Finally, round over your legs to release your spine.

bend the
knees deeply

make the
arms frame
an oval

keep the arms in
line with the back

feel it here

>> **triceps**

7a Holding the weights, stand tall with your legs parallel. Fold at your waist over your legs and tuck your arms in by your sides. Bring your elbows up a little higher than your back. Activate your abs and inhale to begin.

7b Exhale and extend both arms behind you, holding strong in your center. Fold them back in slowly and with control, as though you were pulling something toward you. Repeat 5 more times. Stretch over your legs again before rolling up through your spine, one vertebra at a time.

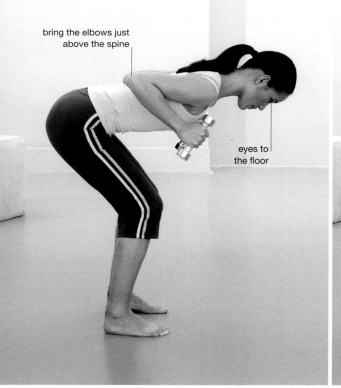

bring the elbows just
above the spine

eyes to
the floor

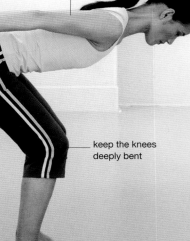

tighten the
triceps

keep the knees
deeply bent

>> **baby circles**

8a Standing in Pilates stance (see p. 19), hold your weights just in front of your legs on a slight angle. Shift your weight toward the fronts of your feet, leaning slightly forward and tightening your gluteal muscles. Begin circling your arms 8 times, raising your arms higher with each circle until you are reaching overhead.

8b Reverse your circles, lowering down for 8 circles. Repeat another full set. Try not to shake or bounce your body as you circle your arms. Hold your torso strong and breathe naturally.

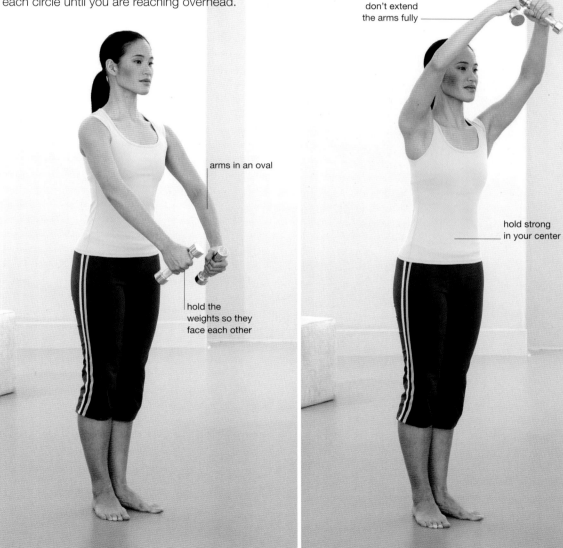

arms in an oval

hold the weights so they face each other

don't extend the arms fully

hold strong in your center

>> lunges

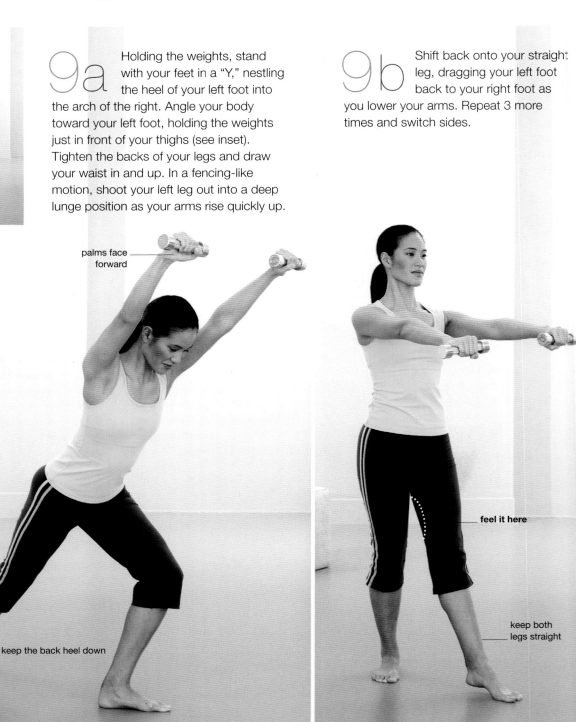

9a Holding the weights, stand with your feet in a "Y," nestling the heel of your left foot into the arch of the right. Angle your body toward your left foot, holding the weights just in front of your thighs (see inset). Tighten the backs of your legs and draw your waist in and up. In a fencing-like motion, shoot your left leg out into a deep lunge position as your arms rise quickly up.

9b Shift back onto your straight leg, dragging your left foot back to your right foot as you lower your arms. Repeat 3 more times and switch sides.

palms face forward

feel it here

keep the back heel down

keep both legs straight

>> **side bend**

10a Stand in Pilates stance and extend your right arm up toward the ceiling, hugging your arm against the side of your head. Inhale and lift even higher, arching up and over to the left.

10b Bend up and away, reaching further over and allowing your bottom arm to hang loosely. Now return to the centerline, resisting on the way up. Lower your arm down by your side and repeat to the left side. Perform 2 more sets for a total of 6 repetitions.

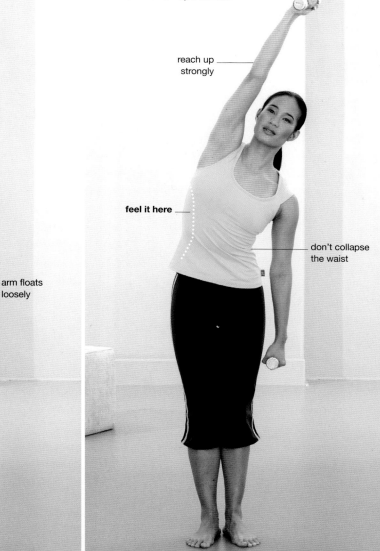

keep the shoulder down

arm floats loosely

reach up strongly

feel it here

don't collapse the waist

>> **push-ups**

11a Stand upright in Pilates stance, tightening the backs of your legs. Reach your arms overhead for a breath, then dive over your legs, reaching for the floor and keeping your abs lifted (see inset). Walk your hands out until you are in a Plank position and bend your knees up.

keep the hips down

keep the hands under the shoulders

11b Open your elbows and lower your upper body up and down for 3 push-ups. Straighten your legs behind you, tuck your toes under, and lift your hips, pressing back into your heels for a stretch. Carefully walk your hands back to your legs, stretch a moment, and roll back up to standing. Repeat 1 more set for a total of 6 push-ups.

tighten the buttocks muscles

keep the neck and head aligned

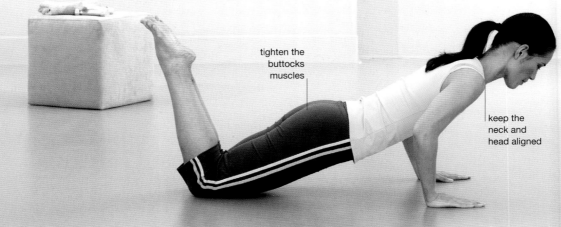

>> **windmill**

12a Stand tall and envision your spine as a wheel as you inhale. Exhale, tucking your head down and folding over your legs. Try to keep your weight shifted slightly forward. Continue exhaling and rounding your spine down in a curling motion.

12b When you are folded over and have no air left, slowly inhale and uncurl your spine, rolling back up to standing. Repeat 2 more times, exhaling progressively longer each time. Finally, roll your shoulders back, lengthen your neck, and stand tall.

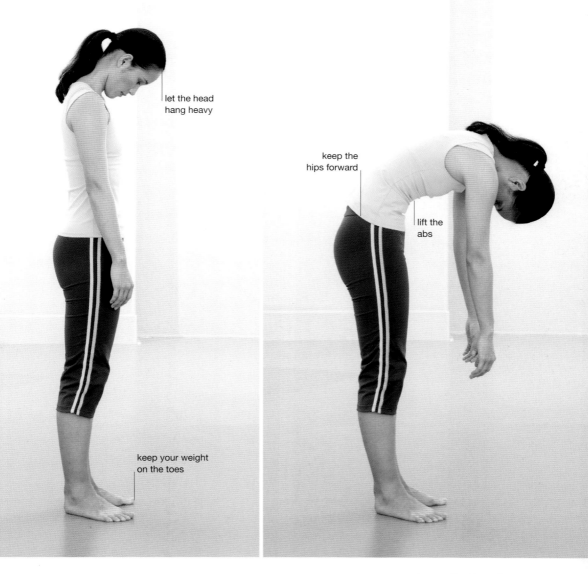

let the head hang heavy

keep the hips forward

lift the abs

keep your weight on the toes

15 minute

Focus on precision
Activate your Pilates stance
Learn the Side Kicks series

from the
bottom up >>

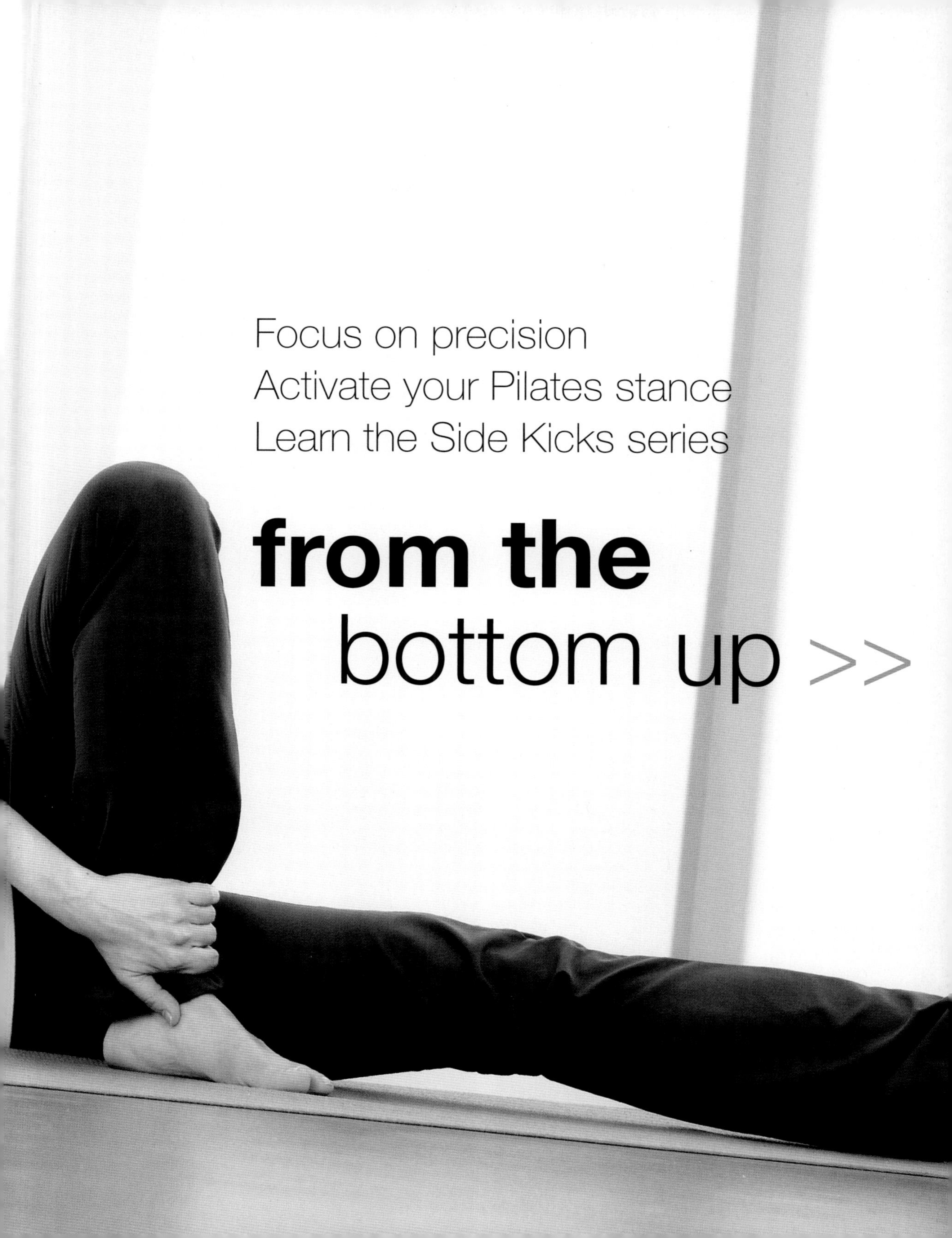

>> pilates stance 1 and 2

keep the
shoulders back

1 Sit tall with your legs in front of you, pressing your inner thighs together and keeping your feet long. Place your hands on the outside of your thighs and squeeze your bottom, rotating your legs and feet so they are slightly open (see inset). Continue to tighten your buttocks muscles, returning your legs and feet to parallel. Perform a total of 5 repetitions.

feel the move with your hands

2 Lie on your back, legs upward, heels together, and toes apart (see inset). Tighten your buttocks and rotate your legs slightly out. Use your hands to cue your muscles to work from your hips. Rotate your legs back to parallel. Repeat 4 more times.

keep the legs together

lift the chest

3a Lie on your right side at the back edge of your mat. Prop your head up with your hand, resting on your elbow, and place your left hand in front of your powerhouse (see p. 19). Keeping your chest lifted (see inset), pull your abs in firmly and lift both legs up in the air, squeezing them tightly.

press the top
shoulder down

squeeze the
backs of the legs

3b Without disrupting your posture, carry your legs forward to the front edge of the mat and lower them with control. You should be at a 45 degree angle on the mat, with your hips and shoulders stacked one on top of the other.

legs at a 45
degree angle

take the elbow to
the back edge of
the mat

>> side kicks front

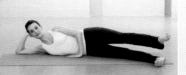

4a Lying on your side at a 45 degree angle on the mat, elevate your left leg and slightly rotate it up to the ceiling. Your right foot remains solidly on the mat, slightly flexed and pressing down into the floor (see inset). Carry your leg forward in a kicking motion, pulsing twice at the height of your kick.

pull the top hip back

don't rotate the bottom leg

4b Sweep your leg down and back behind your body, tightening your buttocks muscles. Keep your upper body still and strong. Repeat a total of 6 times, perfecting your form each time. Bring your leg back to its starting position.

don't lean forward

keep the hips stacked

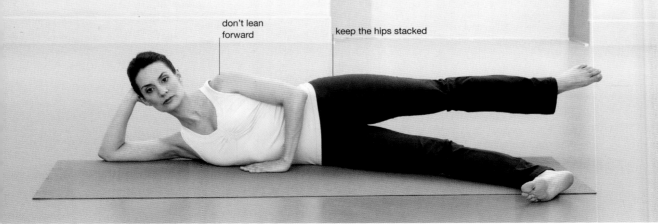

5a Keeping your left leg slightly elevated, rotate it again, turning your foot and knee up to the ceiling. Inhale and kick your left leg high in one swift movement. Aim your leg for a spot just behind your ear as you kick up.

rotate the top leg open

keep the chest high

5b Lower your leg down, creating resistance (see p. 19) as you go, for a count of 3. Use opposition (see p. 19): as your leg lowers, your abs should draw inward and upward. Lift your chest as you repeat 5 more times—for a total of 6 repetitions.

resist as you lower

draw the abs in and up

>> **side kicks circles**

6a Remain lying on your side. Carry your top leg just in front of your bottom leg. It should feel very heavy at this point. Keep it rotated up to the sky with your ankle long.

keep the eyes ahead

keep the front heel facing down

6b Draw 10 tiny circles with your leg in the air without shaking your body. Pause briefly. Switch immediately, taking your left leg back and reversing the circles. Keep the circles tiny and emphasize the downward portion of the circle. Repeat 10 circles and pause before resting your left leg on your right.

keep the shoulders down

feel it here

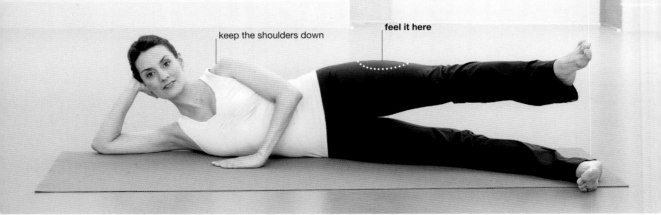

>> side kicks inner-thigh lifts

7a Remain lying on your right side. Cross your left leg in front of your right leg and take hold of your ankle. Place your left foot flat on the floor with your knee and foot pointing down toward your bottom foot. Now, flex your right foot and lift your entire right leg just above the mat.

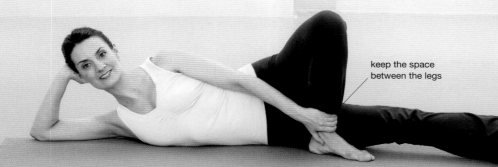

keep the space
between the legs

keep the
foot flexed

7b Without hunching or collapsing, raise your right leg to its highest point and lower it back to above the mat. Repeat 7 more times for a total of 8 repetitions. On the last repetition, remain at the highest point and perfect the position by lengthening, straightening, and rotating just a little bit more. Finally, lower your leg with control.

keep the chest lifted

the foot on the mat angles down

>> **side kicks bicycle**

8a Lie with your legs together at a 45 degree angle in front of you. Raise your left leg slightly. Swing it out in front of your body without hunching or rounding your back (see inset). Create opposition by pulling back, or retracting, your left hip behind you slightly. Bend your left knee in toward your shoulder.

bend the knee in tightly

hold the center strong

8b Sweep your left knee down next to your right knee before extending it behind you. Pull your waist up in opposition to your leg reaching down. Repeat 2 more times and then return your leg to its start position. Reverse direction for 3 more repetitions.

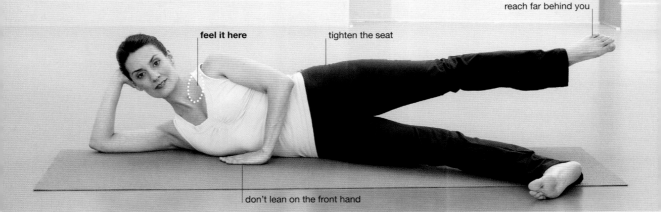

reach far behind you

feel it here   tighten the seat

don't lean on the front hand

9a Transition onto your stomach, then lie face down on your mat. Place your hands under your forehead and stretch your legs out. Tighten your abs and elevate both legs slightly. Keep your shoulders pulling back and down as you open your legs and start to beat them together.

draw the shoulders down

lift the knees off the mat

9b Breathing naturally, continue beating briskly for 20 counts. Beat your legs from the upper inner thighs and keep your knees straight. Pause at the end to lengthen your legs, tighten your abs, and soften your neck and shoulders, before lowering your legs with control. Roll over onto the other side and repeat the Side Kick series (steps 3a–8b) with the opposite leg.

beat the inner thighs together

keep the knees off the floor

>> the teaser

10a

Transition onto your back and bring your knees into your chest as you reach your arms overhead.

keep the ribs in

take the arms in line with the ears

10b

In one count, sweep your body up to sitting, balancing with your legs at 90 degrees, arms reaching forward, abs deeply scooped, chest open. With control, curl your tail under you, laying your spine onto the mat. Fold your knees in, arms overhead to repeat. Perform 5 repetitions.

reach beyond the legs

scoop the abs in

>> the hug

11a

Sit cross-legged with your arms open to the side as though you were holding a weight in each hand. Angle your arms so they slope down from shoulders to elbows to wrists. Press your shoulders down and elongate your neck. Feel that your arms are heavy.

tense the
arm muscles

lengthen the
sides of the waist

11b

Inhale and hug with your arms, creating a huge circle in front of you. Exhale and open your arms with even greater resistance. Repeat 3 times, then reverse your breathing for 3 more repetitions. Keep your abs pulled inward throughout.

keep the
neck long

draw the
shoulders
down

>> **the mermaid**

12a Sit to the right side of your legs with your knees, shins, and ankles stacked on your left. Reach your left hand underneath your bottom ankle and hook onto it, holding firmly. Sweep your free right arm up overhead and inhale to prepare.

lengthen the waist _____

hold the bottom ankle firmly

12b Bend lightly over your legs, exhaling as you stretch your right side. Reach your arm and body higher up as you return to upright. Repeat 2 more times, pausing at the end, lifting your waist, and pulling your shoulders down. Swing your legs to the other side for 3 more repetitions.

reach up and over

open the elbow out

>> **arm circles**

13a Stand in Pilates stance (see p. 19). Shift your weight slightly forward. Hold your arms by your thighs with your palms facing forward (see inset). Inhale, then exhale and raise your arms straight up to the sky.

13b Flip your palms outward and circle your arms down, exerting pressure as though the air were thick. Repeat 2 more times, then reverse the breath, inhaling on the raise and exhaling on the lower, for another 3 repetitions.

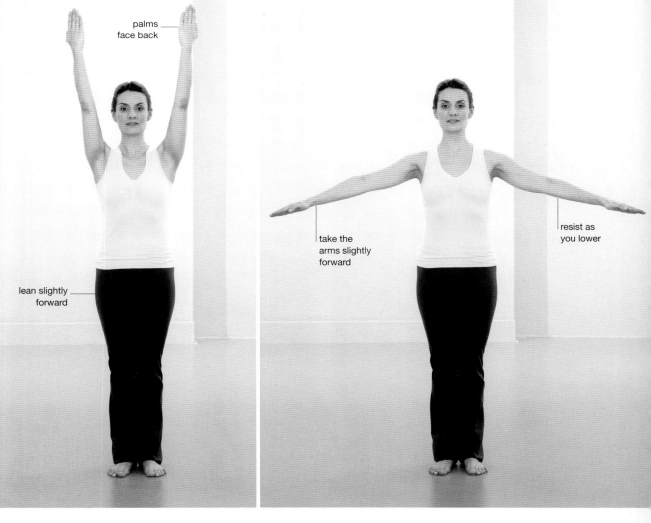

palms face back

lean slightly forward

take the arms slightly forward

resist as you lower

from the bottom up at a glance

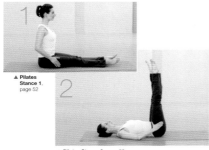

▲ Pilates Stance 1, page 52

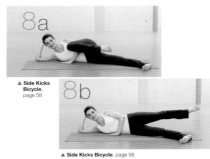

▲ Pilates Stance 2, page 52

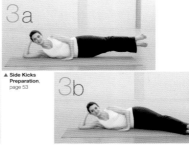

▲ Side Kicks Preparation, page 53

▲ Side Kicks Preparation, page 53

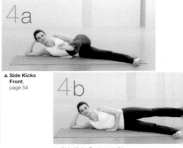

▲ Side Kicks Front, page 54

▲ Side Kicks Front, page 54

▲ Side Kicks Bicycle, page 58

▲ Side Kicks Bicycle, page 58

▲ Beats on Stomach, page 59

▲ Beats on Stomach, page 59

▲ The Teaser, page 60

▲ The Teaser, page 60

up, up, and away at a glance

▲ Neck Press, page 94

▲ Shoulder Roll, page 94

▲ The Hundred, page 95

▲ The Hundred, page 95

▲ Rowing 1, page 96

▲ Rowing 1, page 96

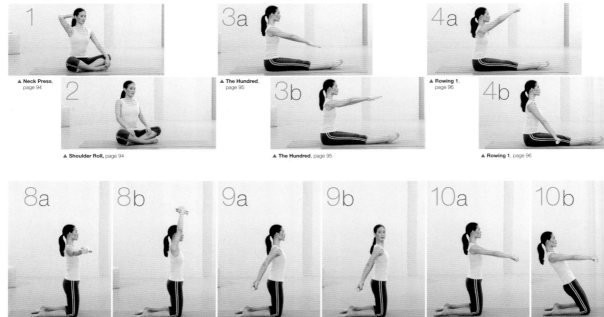

▲ Lotus, page 100

▲ Lotus, page 100

▲ Chest Expansion, page 101

▲ Chest Expansion, page 101

▲ Thigh Stretch, page 102

▲ Thigh Stretch, page 102

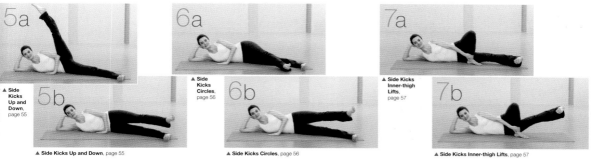

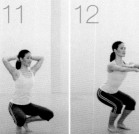

▲ **Side Kicks Up and Down**, page 55

Side Kicks Circles, page 56

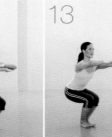

▲ **Side Kicks Circles**, page 56

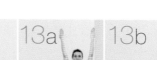

Side Kicks Inner-thigh Lifts, page 57

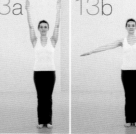

▲ **Side Kicks Inner-thigh Lifts**, page 57

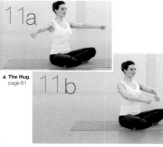

The Hug, page 61

▲ **The Hug**, page 61

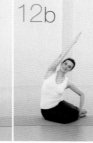

▲ **The Mermaid**, page 62

▲ **The Mermaid**, page 62

▲ **Arm Circles**, page 63

▲ **Arm Circles**, page 63

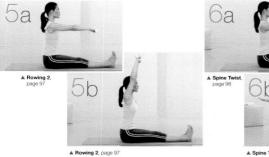

▲ **Rowing 2**, page 97

▲ **Rowing 2**, page 97

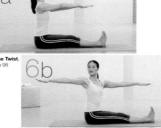

▲ **Spine Twist**, page 98

▲ **Spine Twist**, page 98

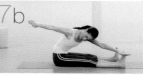

▲ **The Saw**, page 99

▲ **The Saw**, page 99

▲ **Footwork 1**, page 103

▲ **Footwork 2**, page 103

▲ **Footwork 3**, page 104

▲ **Tendon Stretch**, page 104

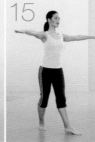

▲ **Front Splits**, page 105

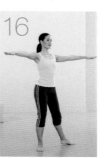

▲ **Side Splits**, page 105

15 minute

Focus on flow
Activate opposition and integration
Learn the standing routine

up, up,
and away >>

>> **neck press/shoulder roll**

keep the
elbow open

1 Sit cross-legged and place one hand behind your head. Draw your chin in and slightly down, thereby pressing your skull back toward your hand. Your neck will lengthen and your waist will draw inward. Meet the resistance of your head with your hand and hold for 3 counts. Release gently. Repeat 4 more times for a total of 5 repetitions.

keep the hips relaxed

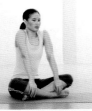

2 With your hands on your knees, inhale and shrug your shoulders forward and up toward your ears (see inset). Then roll your shoulders back, pulling them down as low as they can go, exhaling as you do so. Inhale and repeat 2 more times. Reverse the shoulder circles for 3 more repetitions.

squeeze the
shoulder blades back

hold the abs tight

>> the hundred

3a Sit upright with your legs in front of you. Reach your arms over your legs and draw your waistline in and up. Press your shoulders down firmly and begin pumping your arms briskly up and down, breathing in for 5 counts and out for 5.

sit very tall

keep the abs working

3b Continue pumping as you squeeze your legs and buttocks muscles tight. Hold your body strong so as not to bounce or sway. When you reach 100 pumps or 10 breath cycles, sit taller. Hold for one final moment, then rest.

pump the arms

hold the legs together tightly

>> **rowing 1**

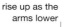

4a Holding the small hand weights, sit tall with your legs extended forward and pressed together. Bend your elbows and pull them behind you to tuck the weights in by your sides (see inset). Inhale and extend your arms up without allowing your shoulders to rise.

press the shoulders down

keep the ankles long

rise up as the arms lower

4b Exhale and lower your arms straight down by your hips. Inhale and lift them up overhead again. Now, reach higher and open your arms sideways, circling them down to begin again. Tuck them in, and repeat twice more for a set of 3 repetitions.

lift the chest high

>> **rowing 2**

5a

Sit tall with your legs extended, feet flexed, and holding the weights by your hips. Inhale and round over your legs. Exhale and press your hands forward along the mat toward your feet (see inset). Keep your abs lifted. Inhale and roll up through your spine to sitting, reaching your arms over your legs.

take the shoulders over the hips

press the heels forward

5b

Continue reaching your arms forward and then take them up to the sky. Circle your arms down and around by your sides to begin again. Repeat a total of 3 times.

circle the arms within your peripheral vision

press the legs together

>> **spine twist**

6a Sit tall with your legs pressed together in front of you and your arms reaching directly over them. Keep your hands reaching long and your feet flexed. Inhale to prepare and lift your waist. Feel the top of your head lengthening up to the sky.

keep the chest lifted

keep the thighs tight

6b Exhale and twist right, taking your right arm backward and rising up in your torso simultaneously. Make another small twist, then rebound to your starting position. Repeat to the left. Perform 4 sets for a total of 8 repetitions, opposing the arms strongly with every twist.

press the back shoulder down

reach the front arm forward

feel it here

feel it here

7a Open your arms side to side, palms face down. Open your legs just past mat width. Flex your feet and lift up tall to begin (see inset). Inhale and twist to the right, keeping your hips and legs planted firmly on the mat.

grow tall as you twist

take the legs hip-width apart

7b Turn your head to follow your back arm. Dive forward, reaching your left hand outside your right foot as though you were sawing off your little toe. Continue to exhale and stretch. Return upright and repeat, twisting to the left. Complete 3 full sets, alternating sides.

let the head hang

feel it here

reach past the little toe

>> lotus

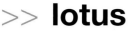

8a Take your weights and kneel upright on your mat with your knees comfortably apart. Your arms extend to the sides of your body with your palms face up. Hold strong in your core and keep your chest lifted.

8b Without disrupting your posture, raise your arms straight up, framing your head and neck in an oval. Lower your arms back down with controlled resistance (see p. 19). Keep your elbows soft. Repeat for a total of 8 times, exhaling to lift and inhaling to lower.

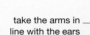

take the arms in line with the ears

keep the arms within your peripheral vision

keep the spine aligned

hold the buttocks tight

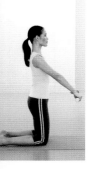

9a Still kneeling upright, hold the weights just in front of you. Tighten your buttocks and pull up in your waist to activate your core. Inhale and sweep your arms behind you with resistance, opening your chest and drawing your shoulder blades together as you go.

9b Keep your arms behind you as you look over your right shoulder and then your left before returning to center. Exhale and take your arms back in front of you. Repeat 3 more times, alternating the initial direction you turn your head with each set.

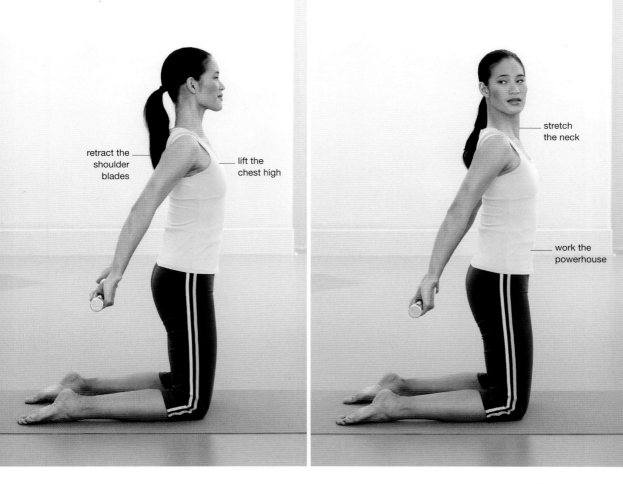

retract the shoulder blades

lift the chest high

stretch the neck

work the powerhouse

>> **thigh stretch**

10a Remain on your knees holding the weights with your arms extended directly in front of you just below shoulder height. Face your palms down and tighten your powerhouse (see p. 19) to begin. Inhale to prepare.

10b Allow your chin to dip down slightly then hinge back, stretching the fronts of your thighs but not arching your spine. At your lowest point, tighten your buttocks and bring your body back up to start again. Perform a total of 4 repetitions, exhaling each time you rise back up. Put the weights down. Tuck your toes under you to come up to standing.

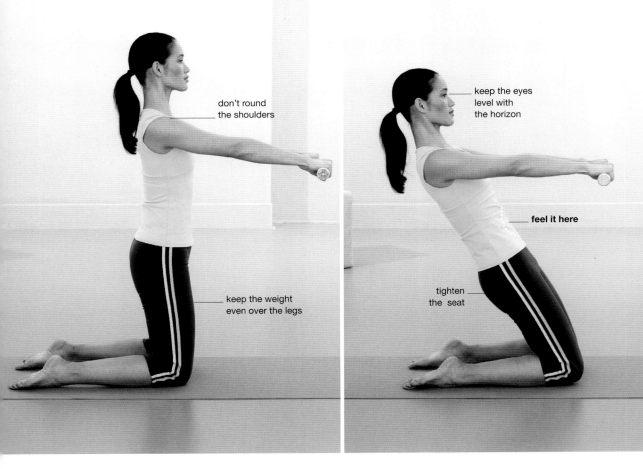

don't round
the shoulders

keep the weight
even over the legs

keep the eyes
level with
the horizon

feel it here

tighten
the seat

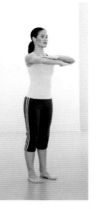

11 Come off your mat and stand up tall in Pilates stance (see p. 19). Place your hands behind your head, elbows wide. Inhale and bend your knees to lower into a squat. Allow your heels to rise. At the bottom of the squat, press your heels into the floor to rise back up. Perform 6 times, inhaling to lower and exhaling to rise.

12 Stand with feet parallel, hip-width apart, arms folded in front of you at chest height. Bend your knees as low as you can go, then push your feet into the floor to rise. Repeat for 6 repetitions. Inhale to lower and exhale to rise.

keep the
spine upright

heels rise
and lower

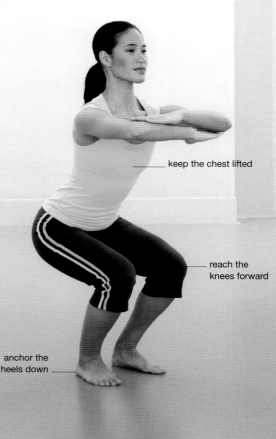

keep the chest lifted

reach the
knees forward

anchor the
heels down

>> footwork 3/tendon stretch

13 Standing with feet together and arms extended in front for stability, curl your toes up and press the rest of your foot firmly down (see inset). Pull your abs in, then bend into a squat. Keep your heels down if possible and stay as upright as you can, resisting the urge to bend too far forward in your spine. Exhale to rise back up with resistance. Don't rush. Repeat a total of 6 times.

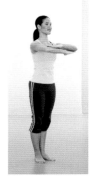

14 Return to Pilates stance, with your arms folded in front at chest height (see inset). Press down firmly into the floor with the balls of your feet so your heels rise up for 3 counts. Lower down with control. Continue for 6 repetitions, exhaling as you rise and inhaling as you lower.

send the hips back

squeeze the inner thighs

lift the toes high

don't lean back

keep the buttocks tight

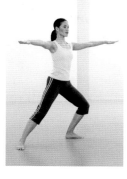

15 Once again, stand in Pilates stance, arms out to your sides. Lunge forward with your left leg, transferring all your weight onto it. Keep your right leg firmly planted into the floor (see inset). Drag your left foot back to the right foot to start again. Inhale to lunge and exhale to pull back 4 times on each leg.

16 Return to Pilates stance, with your arms reaching out to the sides. Lunge sideways with your left leg (see inset), then drag your leg home, straightening it as quickly as possible to activate your upper inner thighs. Repeat 3 more times. Repeat with your other leg to the side.

keep the shoulders down

lift the waist

feel it here

keep the arms within your peripheral vision

make sure the muscles of the inner thighs are working

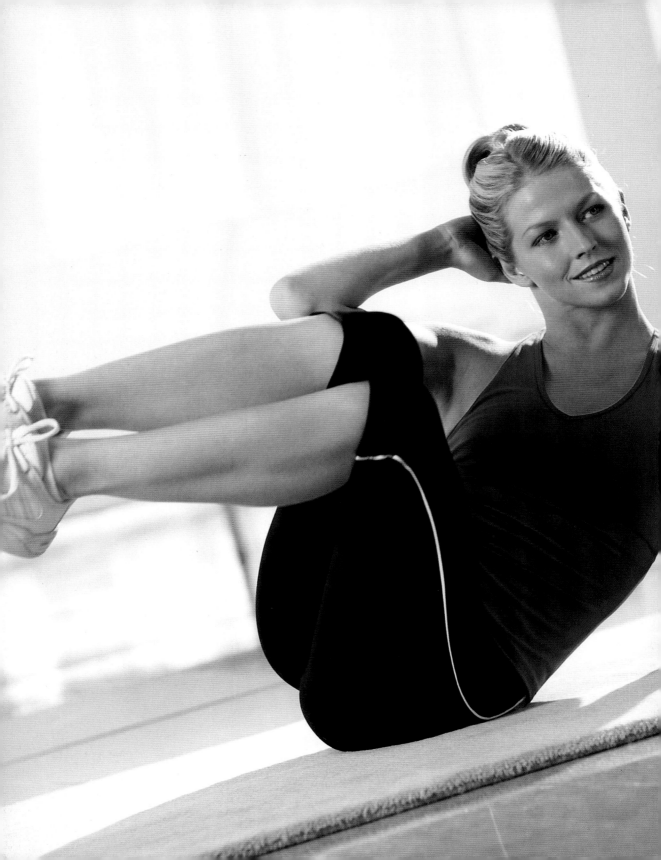

abs
workout

Joan Pagano

>> **focus** on the belly

Walk into any art museum to view the paintings and sculptures, and what do you notice? Women have bellies—it's a fact of nature. There are many factors influencing the size and shape of your belly, but one thing is certain: a healthy lifestyle has a positive effect in every case.

Genetics determine your physical framework, including where you will carry body fat (apple or pear shape). All healthy people have fat reserves necessary for proper functioning of their bodies. Fat tends to accumulate in specific areas, and your personal genetics dictate where you will carry yours. Visceral fat found deep in the abdomen (apple) increases your risk of heart disease, but responds rapidly to diet and exercise.

Differences between the sexes can also play a role. Women typically have a higher percentage of body fat compared to men. This is designed to store the energy needed to nourish a fetus and then a baby. Structurally, a woman's pelvis is tilted a little more forward than a man's so that during pregnancy, there is less pressure on the organs since some of the baby's weight is carried by the abdominal muscles. This anterior tilt of the pelvis gives the impression that the lower belly is slightly pushed out, creating a "pot belly."

Age-related changes occur that affect the shape of our midsection over time. "Middle-aged spread" and "spare tires" typically occur after childbearing as we approach the menopausal years. With advancing age, postural changes can cause spinal curves to become more exaggerated and push the belly forward.

Many other factors may come into play: Weight gain and stress both influence the size of the belly; repeated pregnancies can affect muscle and skin tone; abdominal surgeries can cause a loss of muscle strength, scar tissue, and an accumulation

> ## >> **exercise for** a smaller belly
>
> - **If your abs are toned** but have a layer of belly fat over them, add 30 minutes of cardio most days of the week to burn calories and reduce fat.
>
> - **If you do not have excess belly fat,** but lack of muscle tone causes your belly to hang, you should concentrate on the abs routines to firm up.
>
> - **If you are both** lacking muscle tone and carrying excess fat, step up both cardio (as above) and abs routines. Begin with the Crunch routine.

of fluids. Exercise can help improve many of these.

Before you begin, it is helpful to assess your individual issues and focus on the changes that you can make. Then establish a starting point for your program (see Crunch Assessment, pp. 86–87, Deep Abs Assessment, pp. 88–89, and Safety Issues, pp. 8–9). Set realistic goals and measure your progress periodically.

So many factors influence the size and shape of your belly, including genetic predisposition, age, and lifestyle habits (physical activity and diet).

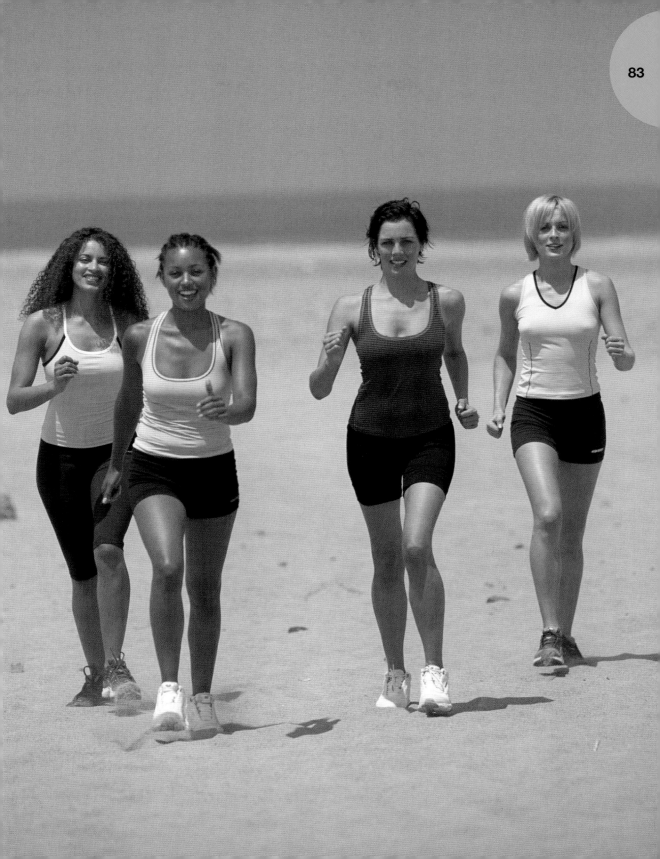

>> **the anatomy** of your abs

The core region of the body is very complex and technically consists of the collective muscles that control your trunk. The abs are central to the core region and work in concert with the erector spinae muscles of the spine to provide stability to the torso.

The abdominals are comprised of four muscle groups: the rectus abdominis, the internal and external obliques, and the transversus abdominis. They are layered, overlapping, and connected to each other. They run vertically, diagonally, and horizontally, and often function synergistically.

The rectus abdominis is best known as the coveted "six-pack" muscle, which describes the

THE CORE MUSCLES

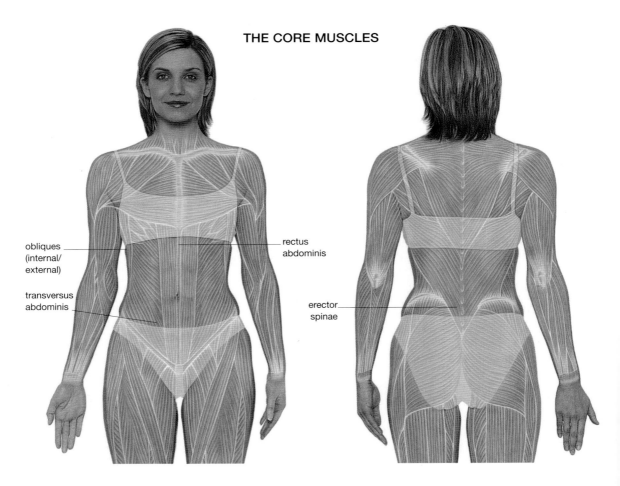

obliques (internal/external)

rectus abdominis

transversus abdominis

erector spinae

sections that develop when this muscle is toned. It is the most superficial muscle of the abdomen, running vertically from the sternum to the pubic bone. It functions to flex the spine and stabilize the pelvis as you walk.

The internal/external obliques are found on the sides of the core area and perform multiple functions. When they contract on one side of the body, they rotate the trunk (see Side Crunch, p. 97), and laterally flex the body (see Side Plank, p. 137). When they contract on both sides of the body simultaneously, they assist in flexing the spine and compressing the abdomen (see Pelvic Tilt, p. 95).

When it is toned, the transversus abdominis acts as a natural girdle, flattening the abdomen and supporting the lower back. It runs horizontally around your midsection and is the deepest abdominal muscle. This muscle works with the internal/external obliques to stabilize the pelvis in a neutral position, as in the 90–90 exercise (see p. 130).

The erector spinae—the spinal extensors—run the length of the spine. Back extensions trigger this group (see Back Extensions, p. 121), strengthening the muscles for greater trunk support. In Plank (see p. 151), the erector spinae functions with the abs to stabilize the torso in the horizontal position.

Like any muscle group, the core muscles require 24 to 48 hours' recovery time between workouts. Although they are primarily endurance muscles, which recover quickly from an abundance of work, they still need time to rest, recover, and rebuild. The result will be added strength.

TARGETING CORE MUSCLES

Do your abs workouts 3 to 4 times a week on nonconsecutive days. Each routine gives you a balanced workout for the abs and spinal muscles. You can do multiple workouts on any given day, but must allow a day of rest before repeating them. The table below shows you which specific muscles are worked by each exercise.

CRUNCH	BEACH BALL	CORE BASICS	CORE CHALLENGE
Rectus abdominis	**Rectus abdominis**	**Rectus abdominis**	**Rectus abdominis**
Short Crunch, p. 95	Roll-back and Lift, p. 113	Roll-back, p. 133	Double Crunch, p. 147
Neutral Crunch, p. 96	Pullover Crunch, p. 115		Crunch and Extend, p. 149
Long Crunch, p. 96	Reverse Crunch Combo, p. 116	**Transversus abdominis**	Kneeling Crunch, p. 151
Diamond Crunch, p. 98		Pelvic Tilt, p. 129	
Reverse Crunch, p. 99	**Transversus abdominis**	Straight-leg Lowering, p. 129	**Transversus abdominis**
90–90 Crunch, p. 100	Reverse Crunch Combo, p. 116	90–90, p. 130	Tuck and Roll, p. 148
Crunch and Dip, p. 100	Toe Tap, p. 118	Alternating Kicks, p. 130	Crunch and Extend, p. 149
Bicycle, p. 101	Ball Transfer, pp. 118-119	Double-leg Lowering, p. 132	Dead Bug, p. 149
			Toe Dip, p. 153
Transversus abdominis	**Obliques**	**Obliques**	
Pelvic Tilt, p. 95	Side Twist, p. 114	Knee Drop, p. 131	**Obliques**
Crunch and Dip, p. 100	Side Reach, p. 115	Spiral Ab Twist, p. 133	Tuck and Roll, p. 148
	Trunk Twist, p. 117	Twisting Roll-back, p. 134	Kneeling Twist, p. 150
Obliques	Balancing Side Crunch, p. 119	Side Plank, p. 137	Kneeling Crunch, p. 151
Side Crunch, p. 97			Twisting Side Plank, p. 152
Torso Twist, p. 99	**Erector spinae**	**Erector spinae**	Balance and Crunch, p. 154
Bicycle, p. 101	Forearm Plank, p. 120	Kneeling Lift, p. 135	
	Back Extension, p. 121	Forearm Plank, p. 135	**Erector spinae**
Erector spinae			Kneeling Crunch, p. 151
Arm and Leg Lift, p. 101			Plank with Leg Lift, p. 151
Press-up, p. 102			Lat Push, p. 156

>> **crunch** assessment

The crunch is the classic abs exercise, targeting the rectus abdominis muscle that runs from the sternum to the pubic bone. It is a versatile exercise, suitable for beginners or more advanced exercisers. It also ranks as one of the most effective for strengthening the abdomen.

The function of the rectus muscle is to flex the spine, and in the crunch you do not perform more than 30 degrees of spinal flexion (which refers to how high you lift your upper torso off the floor), even if you can raise your torso higher. This range of motion isolates the muscle, keeping the work in the rectus. If you lift higher, as in a full sit-up, for example, you activate other muscles, primarily the hip flexors in the front of the thigh. In addition to being a more effective isolation exercise than the full sit-up, the crunch places less stress on the lower back, and is therefore safer.

It is useful to have an objective measure of your starting level of abdominal fitness. Along with your

health and medical information, a fitness assessment helps define your goals in an exercise program. Establishing a baseline also enables you to measure your improvement. One way to measure muscular fitness is to count how many repetitions you can perform. Do the crunch test as described below. Write down your results, make a note of the date, and after two months of training, repeat the assessment.

To get the most from your workout, use proper form and execution of the crunch. Concentrate on perfecting the technique and apply it to each repetition. Mental focus also enhances the outcome: Think about feeling the abdominal muscle tightening, strength coming from the core center, lifting from the chest, head relaxed in your hands.

Preparation for the crunch

Make a cradle for your head by spreading your fingertips and supporting the base of your skull (see p. 87, top right). Bend your fingers slightly and let the weight of your head rest in your hands. Keep your chin lifted, as if you were holding an orange under it (measure the distance with your fist, as in the photograph on p. 87, top left). Keep your elbows wide to reduce any tendency to pull on your neck.

With your lower back relaxed in neutral alignment, engage the rectus abdominis by tightening the connection between the ribs and the hips. Keep tension in the muscle as you lift your chest to the ceiling, shoulder blades clearing

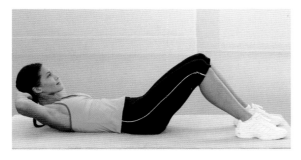

Neutral crunch
Count how many neutral crunches you can do consecutively without resting. Remember, this is not a full sit-up. Lift your shoulders no higher than 30 degrees off of the mat.

Your score

Excellent	50 or more
Good	35–49 reps
Fair	20–34 reps
Poor	fewer than 20 reps

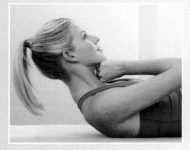

Fist under chin Use your fist under your chin to gauge the correct alignment of the head. Always think: "Chin up."

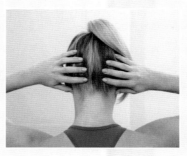

Position of hands on head Spread your fingers at the base of your skull to create a cradle for holding your head. Remember to relax your neck in your hands.

the floor. Maintain the tension as you lower your shoulder blades to the floor, and without resting at the bottom, immediately repeat the lift. Keep drawing the ribs to the pelvis—think of "scooping" out the abdomen. Learn to breathe while you are drawing in, holding tension in the muscle: Inhale first, then exhale as you lift up. Use slow, controlled movements and work the entire range of motion. It's quality not quantity that counts!

The weight of your head and upper torso provide resistance in the

crunch. You can increase the intensity by slowing the action, adding holds (see Long Crunch, p. 96, and Diamond Crunch, p. 98), or by adding external resistance. In Beach Ball (see pp. 106–123), for instance, a simple unweighted ball will do just fine; but you can increase the resistance for muscle strengthening by using a weighted ball of 3–4 pounds (1.4–1.8kg)—my favorite are filled with gel. Although there are heavier balls available, it is better to use one of this weight and maintain proper form, being careful not to use momentum in the movements.

Connecting ribs to hips Set your abs before you move. Think of connecting the ribs to the hips. Maintain this connection, drawing ribs to pelvis, while you perform crunches.

>> **deep abs** assessment

The deepest abdominal, the transversus abdominis, is a flat, horizontal band of muscle that encircles the waist front to back. Toning it creates a natural corsetlike effect of narrowing the waist, flattening the abdomen, and supporting the low back.

The transversus abdominis plays a significant role in core strength. It functions to stabilize the pelvis and maintain the small curve in the lower back, which affects your posture and alignment in all positions against gravity, whether you are stationary or moving. In fitness training, sports activities, and everyday life, a stable core provides stability for the trunk, which increases the control of the movement you are performing.

A few simple exercises can help you to develop body awareness of your deep abdominals. Belly breathing is key here, because the transversus abdominis functions (along with the obliques) to compress the abdomen when you exhale. Practice a belly breath: Inhale, fill the belly with air, then exhale forcefully by pulling the abs tight (think "belly button to spine") and push the air out.

Next, find your own neutral spine alignment, the place where your spine rests while preserving all its natural curves. You should have a slight curve in the lower back—with just enough space to slip your hand in if you are standing straight with your back against a wall. It may be more difficult to establish the neutral position when lying down, but it is halfway between a full arch and a flat-back position. The correct alignment of the lower back, neither flattened nor arched, will allow you to recruit your core muscles most effectively.

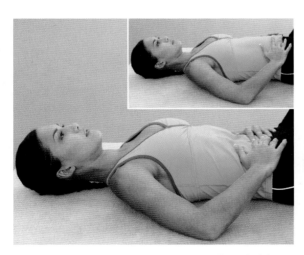

Belly breaths Place your hands on your belly to feel the action of the abs as they expand to take the air in (inset) and compress to push the air out.

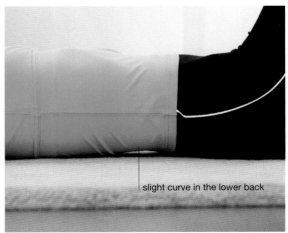

slight curve in the lower back

"Neutral spine alignment" refers to the resting position of the spine with all its natural curves in place. The lower back retains its slight curve and is neither arched nor flattened.

>> tips for **core training**

- **Warm up the pelvis** Do 10 Pelvic Tilts with belly breaths to rehearse the breathing, practice abdominal compression, and move the pelvis in a controlled way.

- **Active stabilization** Do a strong Pelvic Tilt and then release halfway, keeping the abdominals engaged and the lower back relaxed. With the pelvis stabilized like this, breathe naturally.

- **Monitor the position of the pelvis** Place your fingers under your sacrum to make sure it stays level.

The Pelvic Tilt can be used as a technique to learn how to actively stabilize the pelvis in neutral spine alignment. Do a Pelvic Tilt (see p. 95) combining a belly breath with a slight rotation of the pelvis: Inhale, expand the belly as you take in the air; exhale, compress the abdomen, and press the lower back to the floor. Now, keep your abs tight and release the Pelvic Tilt halfway. Relax the lower back, allowing the slight natural curve. The abs should remain taut or stiff to the touch.

To assess the strength of the transversus abdominis, we challenge its ability to stabilize the pelvis against the changing resistance of various leg movements. There are three levels of difficulty, as shown on the right. All variations are performed lying on your back, with your arms resting to the sides, palms up, to minimize any assistance from the upper body. As you add the leg movements, use your abs to keep your lower back from arching and your hips from rocking side to side. A good way to monitor how you are doing is to place your fingers under your pelvis and feel the two bumps on either side of your sacrum just below your waist. As you raise and lower your legs, make sure that the pelvis stays level, exerting even pressure on your fingers, and doesn't lift up on either side.

Assessing the strength of the **transversus abdominis**

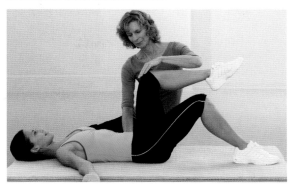

Beginner level Engage the abs, lift one leg at a time, keeping the right angle at the knee, then lower the leg back to the floor. Alternate sides for 10 reps.

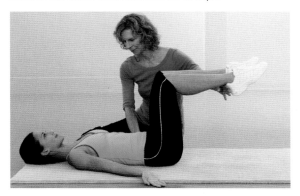

Intermediate level Come into 90–90, one leg at a time, right angles at hips and knees, lower back in neutral alignment. Hold this position for 30 seconds or more.

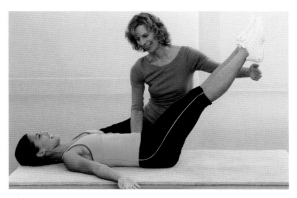

Advanced level From 90–90, straighten both legs to the ceiling and lower them toward the floor, as far as you can without arching the lower back.

15 minute

crunch >>

Shape up with the one of the
most effective ab exercises
Perfect the classic crunch

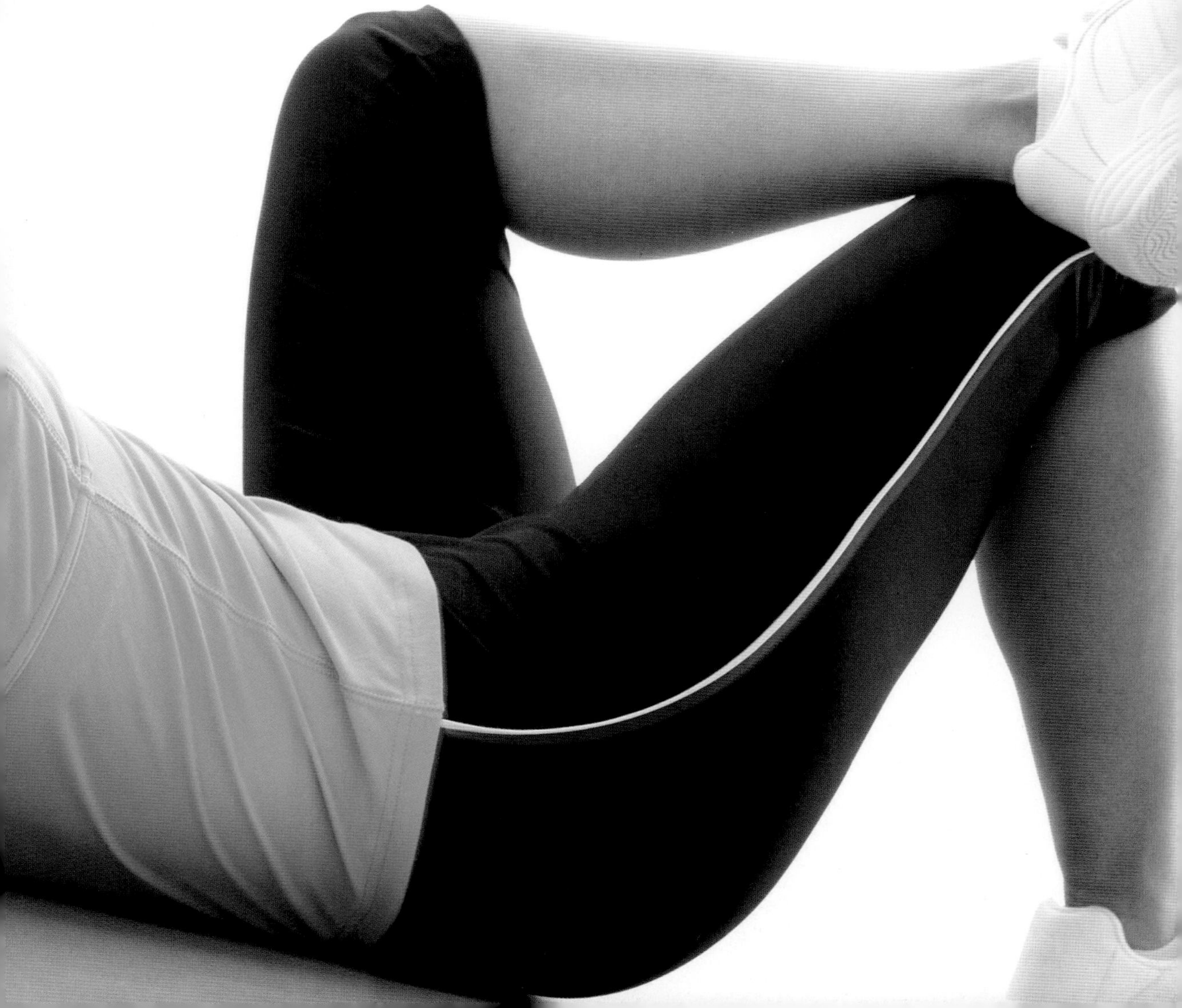

>> march in place/step-touch in

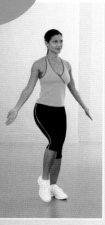

1 To warm up, begin marching with your feet parallel, knees soft, arms by your sides (see inset). Add the arms, lifting them up, then back down. Turn your palms up on the lift, down on the release. March for 16 reps (1 rep = both sides).

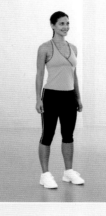

2 Step one leg to the side, arms by your sides (see inset). Step the other leg in, touching your feet together, bending your elbows to that side, and swinging your hands to shoulder height. Repeat, moving from side to side, for 8 reps.

turn the palms down as you lower the arms

keep the knee low

bend the elbows, fists to shoulder height

shift the weight from side to side

3 Step your feet apart, arms by your sides (see inset). Swing both arms to one side at shoulder height, coming up on the toes of the opposite foot. Circle your arms down to the other side and reach out with the tapping leg. Repeat, alternating sides, for 8 reps.

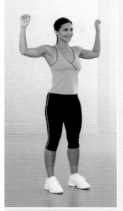

4 With legs apart, raise the arms sideways to shoulder height. Bend your elbows to 90 degrees, palms forward (see inset). Keeping the back straight, bend one knee to hip height. Rotate your torso, bringing the opposite elbow toward the raised knee. Repeat, alternating sides for 8 reps.

arms swing like a pendulum

reach the tapping leg to the side

hold the torso upright

lift the knee to hip height

>> **hamstring curl/body sway**

5 With your legs wider, reach your arms to the sides at shoulder level, palms down (see inset). Bend one knee behind and reach for your foot with the opposite hand, raising the other arm up on a diagonal. Repeat, alternating sides for 8 reps.

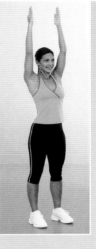

6 With legs apart and arms raised (see inset), step one leg in, flexing at the waist, and head centered between your arms. Repeat, alternating sides for 8 reps. **Repeat steps 5-1** (reverse order) to finish your warm up.

stretch the fingers

reach the hand to the foot

keep the shoulder blades down

the torso and head move as one

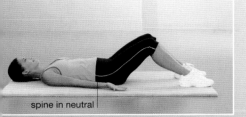

spine in neutral

7 Lie on your back in neutral position with knees bent at 90 degrees, feet flat on the floor, and arms by your sides, palms up. Inhale, filling your belly with air (see inset). Then exhale forcefully, pulling your abs in tight, and with one fluid motion, flatten your lower back to the floor. Hold for a moment, then release and repeat 10 times.

knees bent at 90 degrees

pull the abs tight

arms resting, palms up

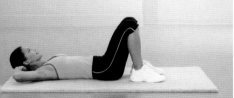

8 From neutral position, move your feet in close to your buttocks, connect the ribs to the hips, then place your hands behind your head (see inset). Inhale first, then exhale, scooping out your abdomen, belly button to spine, as you lift your shoulder blades 30 degrees off the floor. Release, slowly lowering your shoulders (but not your head) to the floor. Repeat 10 times.

keep the chin lifted

feel it here

heels close to the buttocks

>> **neutral crunch/long crunch**

9 Move your feet forward to neutral position. Tighten your abdomen by drawing your ribs toward your pelvis. Pick up the pace and continue to lift and lower your shoulders rhythmically, exhaling as you lift and inhaling as you release, maintaining tension in your abs throughout the movement. Repeat 10 times.

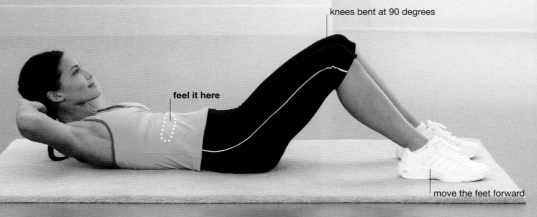

knees bent at 90 degrees

feel it here

move the feet forward

10 Extend your legs, keeping a slight bend in your knees. Inhale first, then exhale and pull *in* when you crunch *up*. Add a hold at the top of the movement and release slowly. Learn to keep tension in the muscle while you continue to breathe. Repeat 10 times, then stretch out, arms and legs long.

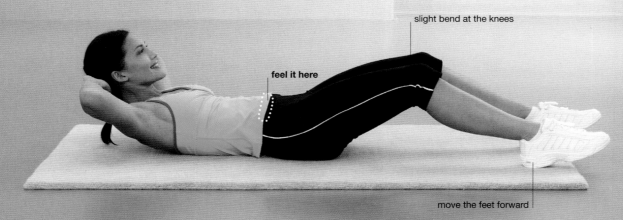

slight bend at the knees

feel it here

move the feet forward

>> **side crunch/lengthening stretch**

11 From neutral position, cross one ankle over the opposite knee, hands behind your head (see inset). With elbows wide, inhale, then exhale and twist one shoulder toward the opposite knee. Pause, then slowly release without resting your head on the floor. Repeat 5 times on each side.

keep the elbows
open wide

feel it here

keep the upper arm of the resting shoulder anchored on the floor

12 Reach out long, extending your arms and legs. Take a deep breath in and stretch out as far as you can. Cross one ankle over the other and take the wrist on the same side in your other hand. Pull to the opposite side, stretching out the entire side of your torso. Pause, then change sides and repeat.

anchor the shoulder blades

crunch >>

>> **bridge/diamond crunch**

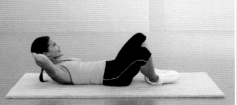

13 Return to neutral position and begin with a Pelvic Tilt (see inset). Then inhale, exhale, and, starting at the base of your spine, peel your back off the floor, one vertebra at a time, until your torso forms a straight line from knees to shoulders. Inhale as you release down, rolling through the curve in your lower back. Repeat 5 times.

torso aligned from the shoulders to the knees

14 Lie with your knees out to the sides, soles of your feet together, as close to your body as possible. Connect your ribs to your hips, then rest your head in your hands and tighten your abs. Exhale as you lift your shoulder blades (see inset). Extend your arms toward your feet, crunching up higher. Return hands behind your head, release down, and repeat 6 times.

crunch higher as you reach

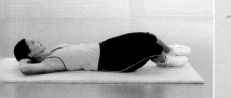

15 Return to neutral position, hands behind head, and bring your legs together, knees and feet touching. Reset your abs. Slowly rotate your pelvis to one side, moving your knees halfway to the floor (see inset). Inhale, then exhale and crunch up toward the ceiling 10 times. Relax your knees to the floor and rest in a Spinal Twist (see p. 114), turning the head in the opposite direction, then repeat to the other side.

feel it here

legs together, knees and feet stacked

knees halfway to the floor

90–90 position

16 Come into 90–90, legs raised with right angles at hips and knees, and arms resting by your sides, palms up (see inset). Inhale, then exhale and pull your belly button in toward your spine, drawing your pelvis toward your rib cage, and lifting your hips. Use control to keep from swinging your legs with momentum. Repeat a total of 10 times.

lift the hips

>> 90–90 crunch/crunch and dip

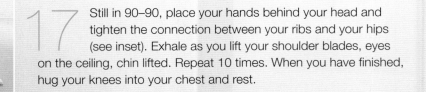

17 Still in 90–90, place your hands behind your head and tighten the connection between your ribs and your hips (see inset). Exhale as you lift your shoulder blades, eyes on the ceiling, chin lifted. Repeat 10 times. When you have finished, hug your knees into your chest and rest.

legs stable at 90–90

shoulder blades clear the floor

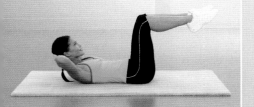

18 Resume 90–90 with your hands behind your head, exhale, and do an upper torso crunch (see inset). Hold it while you inhale and dip your toes to the mat. Exhale and return legs to 90–90, then inhale and release the crunch. Repeat 10 times, then hug your knees into your chest for a breather.

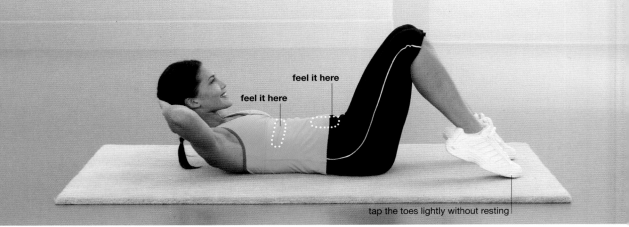

feel it here

feel it here

tap the toes lightly without resting

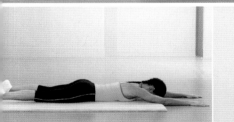

19 Return to 90–90, hands behind your head. Start with an upper torso crunch (see inset), then exhale as you twist one elbow to the opposite knee, bringing your knee into your chest and extending your other leg toward the floor. Inhale back to center and go to the other side. Alternate sides for 5 reps, keeping your shoulder blades lifted. Reach out long to stretch.

twist the shoulder to the knee

feel it here

feel it here

20 Lying face down, extend your arms, palms down. Scoop out your abdomen and press your pubic bone into the floor (see inset). With your forehead still resting, exhale and lift one arm and the opposite leg, lengthening the limbs as you lift up. Repeat for 5 reps.

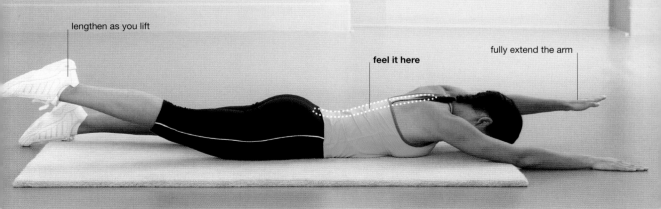

lengthen as you lift

feel it here

fully extend the arm

crunch >>

>> **press-up/sphinx**

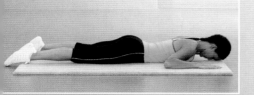

21 Lie face down, arms bent in the shape of a "W," forearms resting on the floor, palms down (see inset). Squeeze your shoulder blades down and together. Lengthen through your torso, reaching the top of your head forward. Exhale as you lift your head and shoulders off the floor without using any strength from your arms. Keep your nose down. Repeat 8 times.

head and neck aligned
with the spine

anchor the shoulder blades

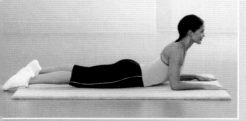

22 Lying face down, elbows bent with forearms resting on the mat, anchor your shoulder blades as you lift your chest, sliding your elbows forward until they are directly under your shoulders. Pull your ribs away from your hips, stretching your abdomen (see inset). With your shoulders square to the front, turn your head to one side and hold; then to the other.

pull the ribs away from the hips

23 Sit back on your heels and bend forward, forehead reaching to mat, arms stretching center (see inset). Walk your hands to one side, keeping your head centered between your elbows, then to the other side. Use your breath to deepen the stretch: let your body sink into the position with every exhale.

head centered
between the
elbows

24 Kneel on all fours, wrists under shoulders, knees under hips (see inset). From neutral, lift your head and hips up, curving your spine into a "C."

lift the hips up

lift the head up

crunch >>

25 Now arch your spine, rounding your back up to the ceiling by tucking your hips under and dropping your head between your arms. Repeat each curve and arch 4 times, breathing naturally throughout.

tuck the hips under

drop the head between the arms

26 Sit up tall, hips firmly planted on the floor, legs crossed comfortably in front. Anchor your shoulder blades. Tilt your ear to your shoulder, using your hand on the side of your head to gently deepen the stretch, while you reach down with your other hand to create a dynamic opposition. Hold and breathe.

tilt the ear to the shoulder

reach down with the opposite hand

pull the top of the head down

turn the chin to the armpit

27 From the previous position, turn your chin to your armpit and place your hand on the crown of your head using gentle downward pressure. Feel a slight shift in the muscles being targeted, now in the back of your neck and upper back. Hold, breathe, and then switch sides, repeating both stretches.

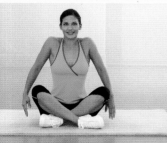

roll the shoulders backward

28 Initiate the movement from your shoulder blades. First shrug them up toward your ears (see inset), then roll them back and together. Then separate the blades as your shoulders come forward and repeat once more. Rolling your shoulders backward will leave your chest open.

crunch >>

crunch at a glance

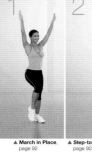
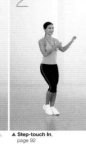
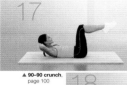
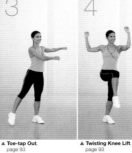
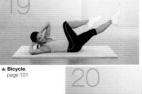
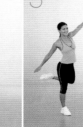
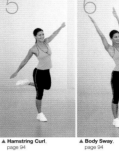
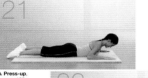
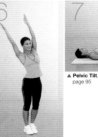
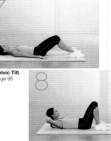

▲ **March in Place**, page 92

▲ **Step-touch In**, page 92

▲ **Toe-tap Out**, page 93

▲ **Twisting Knee Lift**, page 93

▲ **Hamstring Curl**, page 94

▲ **Body Sway**, page 94

▲ **Pelvic Tilt**, page 95

▲ **Short Crunch**, page 95

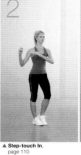
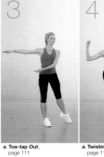
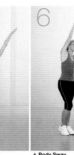
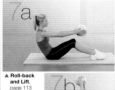

▲ **90–90 crunch**, page 100

▲ **Bicycle**, page 101

▲ **Press-up**, page 102

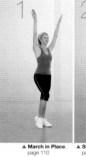
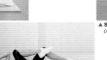
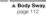
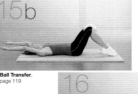
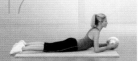

▲ **Crunch and Dip**, page 100

▲ **Arm and Leg Lift**, page 101

▲ **Sphinx**, page 102

beach ball at a glance

▲ **March in Place**, page 110

▲ **Step-touch In**, page 110

▲ **Toe-tap Out**, page 111

▲ **Twisting Knee Lift**, page 111

▲ **Hamstring Curl**, page 112

▲ **Body Sway**, page 112

▲ **Roll-back and Lift**, page 113

▲ **Roll-back and Lift**, page 113

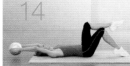
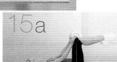
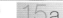

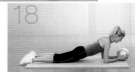

▲ **Toe Tap**, page 118

▲ **Ball Transfer**, page 119

▲ **Sphinx**, page 120

▲ **Ball Transfer**, page 118

▲ **Balancing Side Crunch**, page 119

▲ **Forearm Plank**, page 120

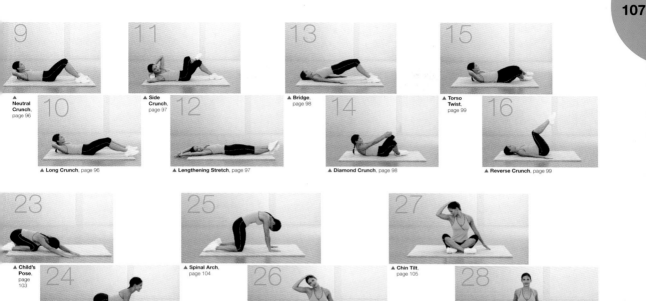

9

10

▲ Neutral Crunch, page 96

▲ Long Crunch, page 96

11

12

▲ Side Crunch, page 97

▲ Lengthening Stretch, page 97

13

14

▲ Bridge, page 98

▲ Diamond Crunch, page 98

15

16

▲ Torso Twist, page 99

▲ Reverse Crunch, page 99

23

24

▲ Child's Pose, page 103

▲ Spinal Curve, page 103

25

26

▲ Spinal Arch, page 104

▲ Ear Tilt, page 104

27

28

▲ Chin Tilt, page 105

▲ Shoulder Roll, page 105

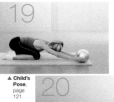

8

9

▲ Side Twist, page 114

▲ Spinal Twist, page 114

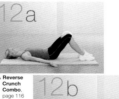

10

11

▲ Pullover Crunch, page 115

▲ Side Reach, page 115

12a

12b

▲ Reverse Crunch Combo, page 116

▲ Reverse Crunch Combo, page 116

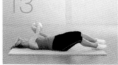

12c

13

▲ Reverse Crunch Combo, page 117

▲ Trunk Twist, page 117

19

20

▲ Child's Pose, page 121

▲ Back Extension, page 121

21

22

▲ Bridge Stretch, page 122

▲ Lower-back Stretch, page 122

23

24

▲ Seated Spinal Twist, page 123

▲ Forward Bend, page 123

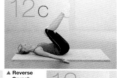
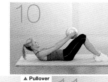
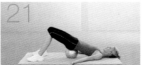
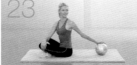
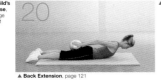
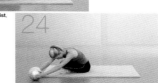
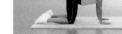
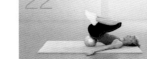

15 minute

beach ball >>

Use a ball to add fun and resistance
Give new energy to traditional exercises

>> march in place/step-touch in

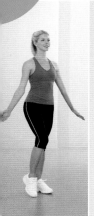

1 To warm up, begin marching with your feet parallel, knees soft, and arms by your sides (see inset). Add the arms, lifting them up, with palms up, then down, with palms down. March for 16 reps (1 rep = both sides).

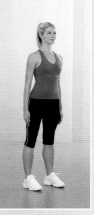

2 Step one leg to the side, arms by your sides (see inset). Step the other leg in, touching your feet together, bending your elbows to that side, and swinging your hands to shoulder height. Repeat, moving from side to side, for 8 reps.

turn the palms down as you lower the arms

keep the knee low

bend the elbows, fists to shoulder height

shift the weight from side to side

3 Step your feet apart, arms by your sides (see inset). Swing both arms to one side at shoulder height, coming up on the toes of the opposite foot. Circle your arms down to the other side and reach out with the tapping leg. Repeat, alternating sides for 8 reps.

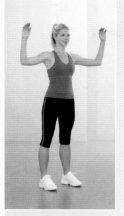

4 With legs apart, raise the arms sideways to shoulder height. Bend your elbows to 90 degrees, palms forward (see inset). Keeping the back straight, bend one knee to hip height. Rotate your torso, bringing the opposite elbow toward the raised knee. Repeat, alternating sides for 8 reps.

arms swing like a pendulum

hold the torso upright

lift the knee to hip height

reach the tapping leg to the side

>> hamstring curl/body sway

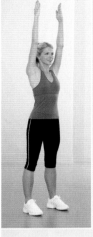

5 Take your legs wider and reach your arms out to the sides at shoulder level, palms down (see inset). Bend one knee behind and reach for your foot with the opposite hand, raising the other arm up on a diagonal. Repeat, alternating sides for 8 reps.

6 With legs apart and arms raised, step one leg in and flex at the waist. Keep your head centered between your arms (see inset). Repeat, alternating sides for a total of 8 reps. **Repeat steps 5-1** (reverse order) to complete your warm up.

stretch
the fingers

keep the
shoulder blades
down

torso and
head move
as one

reach the hand
to the foot

7a Sit tall, knees bent at 90 degrees, hip-width apart, feet flat on the mat. Hold the ball in front of your chest, arms extended. With your spine straight, pull your torso as close to your thighs as you can (see inset). Inhale, then exhale as you roll back, drawing your ribs to your hips, and curling your pelvis under. Think of curving your spine into a "C."

draw the ribs
to the hips

curve the spine,
pull the abs tight

7b Hold the position as you lift the ball overhead, then lower it and realign your spine to straighten up. Repeat 10 times.

keep the shoulder
blades down as
you lift the ball up

8 Sit up with your knees bent at 90 degrees, feet relaxed. Hold the ball close to your body, elbows bent. Lean back with your spine straight, chest lifted (see inset). Rotate your torso to one side and touch the ball to the floor. Then pause at center before repeating to the other side. Repeat for 10 reps.

keep the back straight

touch the ball to the floor

9 Roll down to the floor, keeping your knees bent, and set the ball aside. Stretch your arms out at shoulder level, with your palms facing up, and rotate your knees to one side in a Spinal Twist. Turn your head the opposite way. Hold for a moment, then change sides.

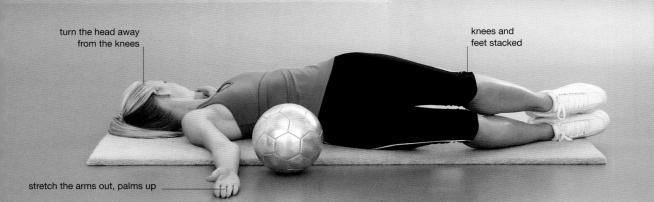

turn the head away from the knees

knees and feet stacked

stretch the arms out, palms up

>> **beach ball**

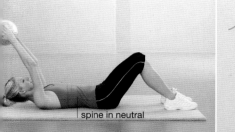

spine in neutral

10 Lie on your back in neutral position, knees bent at 90 degrees, and feet flat on the floor. Hold the ball diagonally overhead with your shoulder blades anchored (see inset). Inhale, then exhale, keep your abs tight, and lift your torso, reaching the ball to your knees. Release back without resting and repeat 10 times. Then rest and rock your head from side to side.

chin up, head and
neck aligned

11 Lie on your back in the neutral position. Hold the ball toward your knees, arms straight (see inset). Inhale, then exhale and lift your shoulder blades, reaching the ball to one side. Hold. Pass through center to the other side. Repeat for 8 reps, alternating sides. Finally, extend your legs and reach your arms long, with the ball behind your head. Rock your head from side to side to ease any tension in the neck.

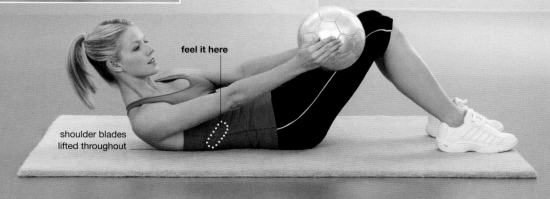

feel it here

shoulder blades
lifted throughout

>> **reverse crunch combo**

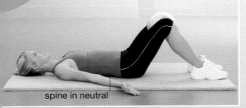

spine in neutral

12a Place the ball between your knees and come into neutral position, arms by your sides, palms up (see inset). To initiate the Bridge, perform a Pelvic Tilt (see p. 95).

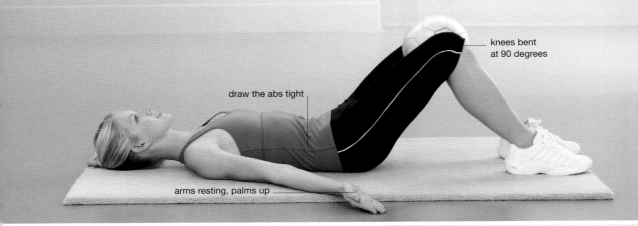

knees bent at 90 degrees

draw the abs tight

arms resting, palms up

12b Complete the Bridge by lifting your hips until they form a straight line connecting your knees to your shoulders. Release, rolling down sequentially through your spine.

straight line from the shoulders to the knees

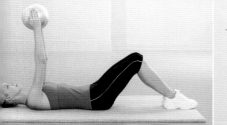

90–90 position

do a Pelvic Tilt as you lift the hips up

shoulder blades anchored to keep the shoulders open

12c Then immediately initiate the Reverse Crunch by raising your legs to 90–90, knees over hips, calves parallel to the floor (see inset). Repeat the Pelvic Tilt, compressing your abdomen and lifting your hips off the floor in a slow controlled movement. Continue, alternating the Bridge and Reverse Crunch for 8 reps (1 rep = Bridge/Reverse Crunch).

13 From neutral position, bring your legs together, knees and ankles touching. Reach the ball toward the ceiling over your chest (see inset). Lower your knees to one side while you reach the ball to the other. Keep your knees and feet stacked as you rotate your pelvis. Repeat for 8 reps, alternating sides. Now set the ball down and do a Spinal Twist (see p. 114) to each side.

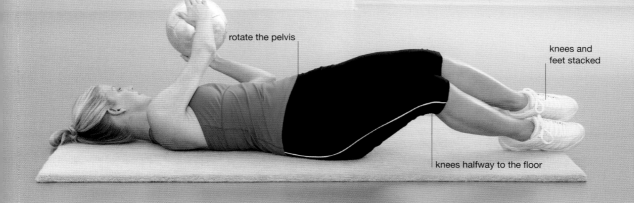

rotate the pelvis

knees and feet stacked

knees halfway to the floor

>> toe tap/ball transfer

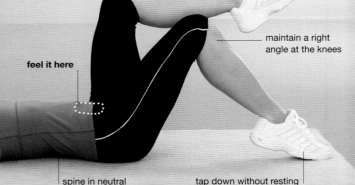

14 Hold the ball above your chest, arms straight, and take your legs to 90–90. Contract your abs to bring your spine into neutral (see inset). Inhale, lowering the ball behind your head as you lower one leg to the floor, maintaining the right angle at the knee. Tap your toes lightly without resting and exhale to return to the starting position. Alternate sides for 6 reps.

maintain a right
angle at the knees

feel it here

spine in neutral   tap down without resting

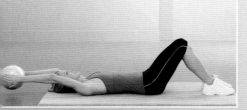

15a In neutral position, hold the ball behind your head, shoulder blades down. Engage your abs to stabilize your upper pelvis against the floor (see inset). Inhale first, then, keeping your head and shoulders on the floor, exhale and raise your arms and legs to place the ball between your knees.

legs at 90–90

head and
shoulders resting

15b Inhale, lowering your arms and feet toward the floor without arching your back. Tap toes down, then exhale as you lift your limbs again to grasp the ball in your hands and return to the starting position. This is 1 rep. Repeat steps 15a and 15b for a total of 5 reps, then stretch out long, holding the ball behind your head.

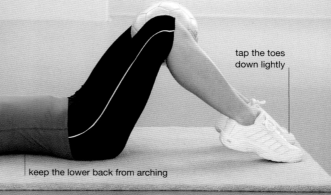

tap the toes down lightly

keep the lower back from arching

16 In neutral position, place the ball under one foot and extend the other leg (see inset). With the hands behind the head and the elbows wide, exhale and lift the shoulder blade, twisting that shoulder toward the knee as the working leg bends to meet the elbow. Do this 10 times. Change sides and repeat.

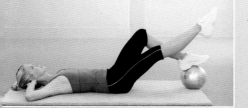

push through the heel to stabilize the leg on the ball

keep the upper arm anchored on the floor

>> sphinx/forearm plank

17 Turn onto your stomach and draw your shoulder blades down and together. Lift your chest, position your elbows directly under your shoulders, and hold the ball between your hands. Reach the top of your head toward the ceiling while you breathe into the stretch, lengthening through the torso.

draw the shoulder blades down and together

press the pubic bone into the floor

elbows under the shoulders

18 From the Sphinx, with your shoulders anchored and still holding the ball, scoop out your abs and lift your hips, making a straight line from shoulder to knee. Keep your shoulder blades wide and apart, head and neck aligned with your spine. To increase the intensity of the exercise, tuck your toes under and lift your knees.

lift the hips

draw the abs tight

relax the hands on the ball

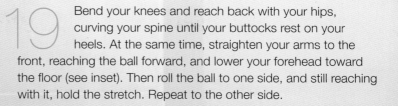

19 Bend your knees and reach back with your hips, curving your spine until your buttocks rest on your heels. At the same time, straighten your arms to the front, reaching the ball forward, and lower your forehead toward the floor (see inset). Then roll the ball to one side, and still reaching with it, hold the stretch. Repeat to the other side.

keep reaching
for the ball

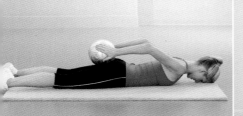

20 Holding the ball with both hands, slide forward onto your stomach, legs hip-width apart. Move the ball to your lower back, holding it with fingers pointing back, elbows bent to the ceiling (see inset). Rest your forehead on the mat. Inhale, then exhale, lift your chest and straighten your arms, pressing the ball down your back. Inhale and bend your arms to return. Repeat 10 times.

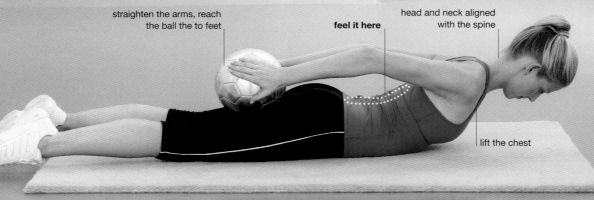

straighten the arms, reach
the ball the to feet

feel it here

head and neck aligned
with the spine

lift the chest

>> bridge stretch/lower-back stretch

21 Turn onto your back, knees bent, feet on the floor. Lift your hips and place the ball under your sacrum, allowing it to support your body weight. Inhale, and on the exhale feel the lower back relax. Hold the ball with your hands, if necessary. Take several deep breaths.

body weight rests on the ball

22 From the Bridge stretch, bring one knee up over your chest and then the other. Separate the knees, still allowing the ball to support you. Continue to hold onto the ball or turn your palms up and rest your arms by your sides. With every exhale, let your body weight sink into the ball. To come out of the stretch, hold onto the ball and lower one leg at a time.

relax the lower back

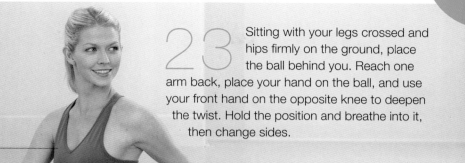

23 Sitting with your legs crossed and hips firmly on the ground, place the ball behind you. Reach one arm back, place your hand on the ball, and use your front hand on the opposite knee to deepen the twist. Hold the position and breathe into it, then change sides.

sit up straight

use the hand on the opposite knee

keep the hips firmly planted

24 Return to center and bring the ball to the front. With your sitbones anchored on the floor, bend forward, rounding your spine, and reaching the ball to the front with your arms straight. Breathe into the stretch (see inset). Then roll the ball to one side, torso facing your knee, and hold. Repeat on the other side and return to center.

the ball extends your reach

sitbones are down evenly

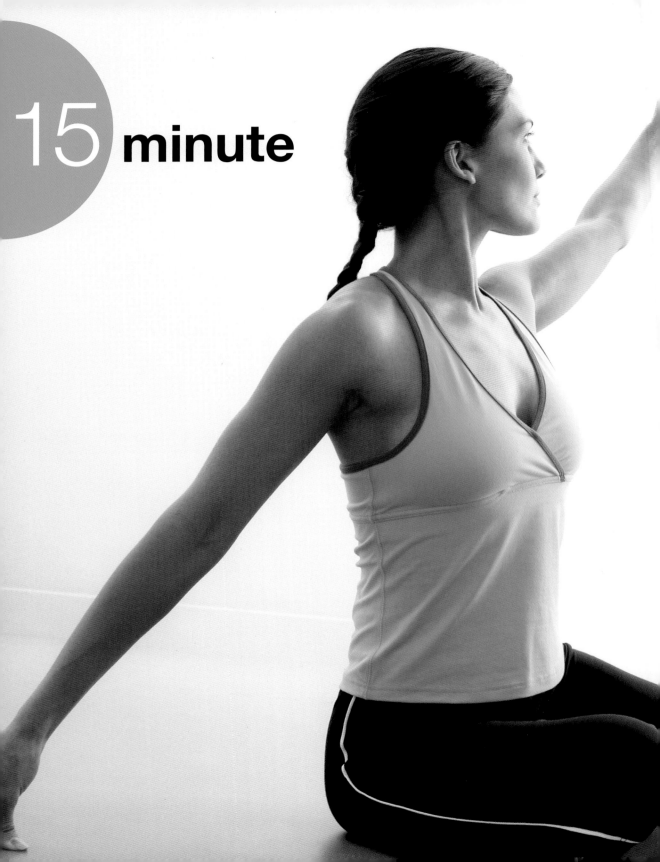

15 minute

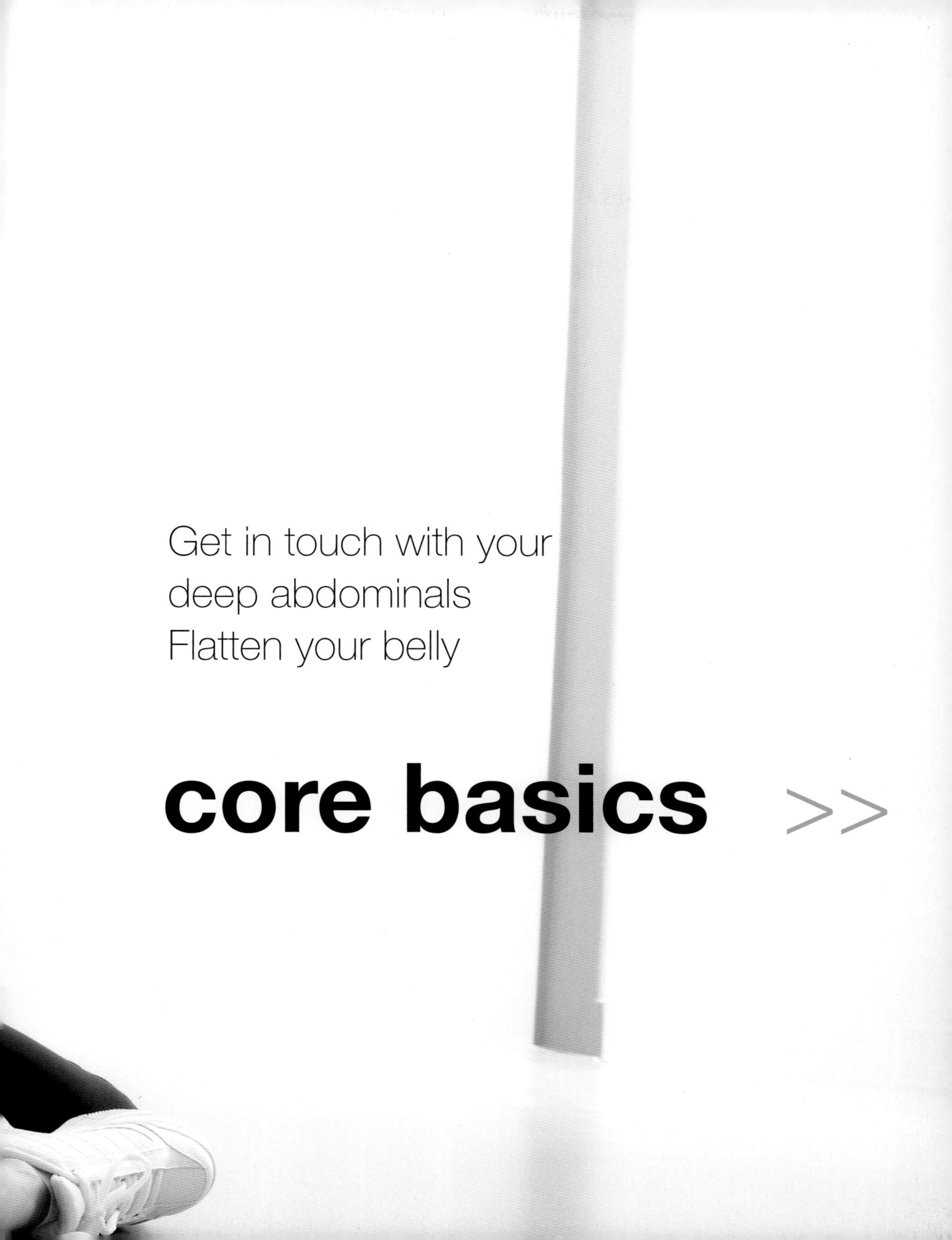

Get in touch with your
deep abdominals
Flatten your belly

core basics >>

>> march in place/step-touch in

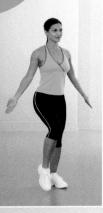

1 To warm up, begin marching with your feet parallel, knees soft, and arms by your sides (see inset). Add the arms, lifting them up, then back down. Turn your palms up on the lift, down on the release. March for 16 reps (1 rep = both sides).

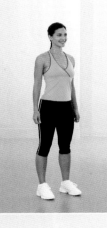

2 Step one leg to the side, arms by your sides (see inset). Step the other leg in, touching your feet together, bending your elbows to that side, and swinging your hands to shoulder height. Repeat, moving from side to side, for 8 reps.

turn the palms down as you lower the arms

keep the knee low

bend the elbows, fists to shoulder height

shift your weight from side to side

>> toe-tap out/twisting knee lift

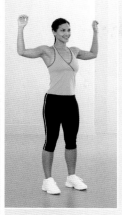

3 Step your feet apart, arms by your sides (see inset). Swing both arms to one side at shoulder height, coming up on the toes of the opposite foot. Circle your arms down to the other side and reach out with the tapping leg. Repeat, alternating sides for 8 reps.

4 With legs apart, raise the arms sideways to shoulder height. Bend elbows to 90 degrees, palms forward (see inset). Keeping the back straight, bend one knee to hip height. Rotate your torso, bringing the opposite elbow toward the raised knee. Repeat, alternating sides for 8 reps.

arms swing like a pendulum

reach the tapping leg to the side

hold the torso upright

lift the knee to hip height

>> **hamstring curl/body sway**

5 Take your legs wider and reach your arms sideways at shoulder level, palms down (see inset). Bend one knee behind you and reach for your foot with the opposite hand, raising the other arm up on a diagonal. Repeat, alternating sides for 8 reps.

stretch the fingers

reach the hand to the foot

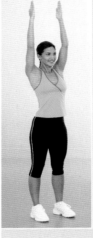

6 With legs apart and arms raised, step one leg in, flexing at the waist and head centered between your arms (see inset). Repeat, alternating sides for 8 reps. **Repeat steps 5-1** (reverse order) to complete your warm-up.

keep the shoulder blades down

torso and head move as one

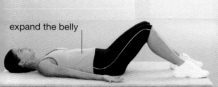

expand the belly

7 Lie in neutral position, knees bent at 90 degrees, hip-width apart, with feet flat on the floor. Rest your arms by your sides, palms up. Begin with a belly breath (see inset), then exhale forcefully, compress your abdomen, and rotate your pelvis backward, pressing your lower back to the floor. Hold for a moment, then release. Repeat for 10 reps.

compress the abs

press the lower back to the floor

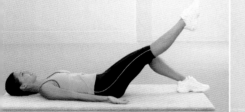

8 In neutral position, do a strong Pelvic Tilt and release halfway so your lower back goes into its natural curve. Keep your abs tight to stabilize your pelvis in this position. Extend one leg to the height of the other knee (see inset). Inhale and slowly lower the leg toward the floor; exhale and return to start. Repeat 6 times, then change sides.

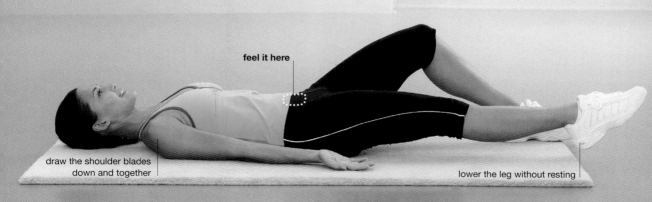

feel it here

draw the shoulder blades down and together

lower the leg without resting

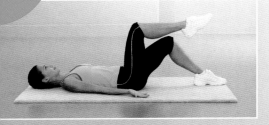

9 Begin in neutral position. Reposition the Pelvic Tilt and release halfway, keeping your abs engaged. With your pelvis stabilized, bring one knee up over your hip (see inset) and then the other, keeping your calves parallel to the floor. Hold this 90 degree angle at both the hip and the knee. You should feel strain in your lower abs.

knees over the hips

calves parallel to the floor

10 From 90–90, bring one knee in over your chest and straighten the other leg, lowering it as close to the floor as possible without arching your back. Pause, then return to the starting position and repeat, alternating legs for 5 reps. When you're done, hug your knees into your chest and rock from side to side.

bring the knee over the chest

lengthen the leg toward the floor

11 Come into 90–90, abs strong, pelvis stable, arms resting by your sides, and palms up. Press your knees and feet together (see inset). Inhale as you rotate your pelvis to one side, lowering your knees halfway to the floor. Exhale and return to center. Continue, alternating sides, for 6 reps.

tighten the abs as you rotate the pelvis

legs together, knees and ankles stacked

12 Bring your feet to the floor in neutral position, then rotate your knees to one side. Stretch your arms out to the sides at shoulder level, palms up. Rest, turning your head to the opposite side. Hold the position briefly and breathe, then change sides.

stretch the arms out at shoulder level, palms up

>> **double-leg lowering**

bend the legs at 90–90

13a Return to 90–90, arms by your sides and palms up to keep your shoulders open (see inset). Extend both legs to the ceiling and point your toes. Draw your abs in tight to stabilize the top of your pelvis against the floor, lower back in neutral position.

extend the legs to the ceiling

13b Exhale as you lower both legs toward the floor, going as far as you can without arching your lower back. Keep pulling your abs in as you go. Inhale, bend your knees in, and return to start. Repeat 10 times. Hug your knees in to rest.

keep the legs together

feel it here

lower the legs without arching your back

press the arm back

14 Sit on one hip, legs bent to the other side, front foot aligned with the opposite knee. Plant your supporting hand on the ground in line with your shoulder and extend your other arm up on a diagonal. Look up at your hand. Inhale and press your raised arm back to stretch your torso (see inset). Exhale, contract your abs, and curl the raised arm under the supporting arm. Repeat 8 times, then change sides and repeat 8 times.

feel it here

curl the shoulder in, reach the arm through

feel it here

15 Sit up straight, knees bent at 90 degrees, feet flat. Pull your torso in close to your thighs. Reach your arms forward at shoulder level, palms down (see inset). Exhale, and take your belly button to your spine, as you roll back onto your tailbone. Inhale and realign your spine to straighten up. If you need help, use your hands on your thighs. Repeat for 4 reps.

feel it here

curve the spine, ribs to hips

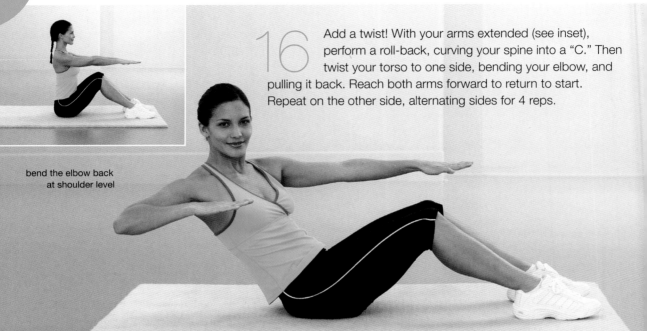

16 Add a twist! With your arms extended (see inset), perform a roll-back, curving your spine into a "C." Then twist your torso to one side, bending your elbow, and pulling it back. Reach both arms forward to return to start. Repeat on the other side, alternating sides for 4 reps.

bend the elbow back
at shoulder level

17 Holding onto your thighs, roll down to the floor and extend your arms and legs. Take a deep breath in and stretch out as far as you can. Exhale and relax. Cross one ankle over the other and take the wrist on the same side in your other hand. Pull to the opposite side, creating a stretch down one side of your body. Repeat on the other side.

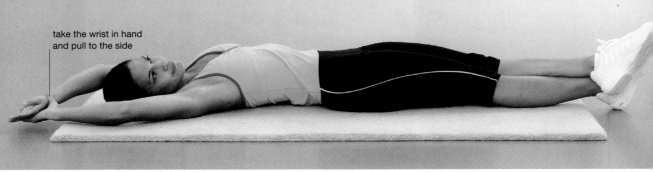

take the wrist in hand
and pull to the side

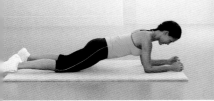

18 Kneel on all fours, wrists under shoulders, knees under hips. Extend one leg to hip height, then lift the opposite arm to shoulder level. Stabilize the supporting arm by spreading your fingers and pushing into your thumb and index finger (see inset). Hold, then lower and lift your limbs 6 times and hold again. Repeat on the other side.

touch down lightly without resting

19 From the kneeling position, take your hands forward and place your forearms on the floor, elbows directly under your shoulders. Take your knees back and drop your hips, creating a straight line from shoulder to knee. Pull your abs in tight, and anchor your shoulder blades (see inset). Hold, then straighten your legs and come onto your toes in the full forearm plank position. Hold.

anchor the shoulder blades

tuck the toes under

elbows under the shoulders

>> forearm plank plus/child's pose

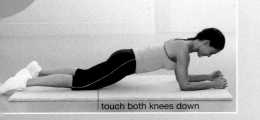

touch both knees down

20 From the full Plank, lower both knees simultaneously 4 times (see inset). Then lower one knee at a time, alternating sides for 4 reps. If you are fatiguing, just try to hold the Forearm Plank from the knees. Breathe naturally throughout.

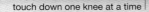

keep the hips level

touch down one knee at a time

21 Sit back into Child's Pose, with your hips to your heels and your forehead to the floor. Stretch your arms forward. Take a few seconds to rest in this position and refresh yourself. Breathe deeply, releasing tension from your muscles with every exhale.

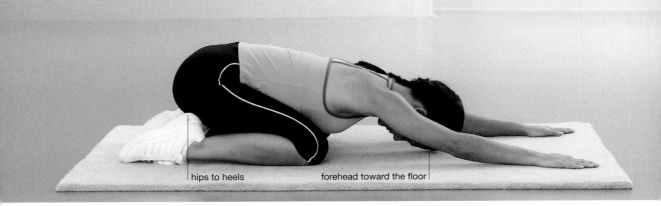

hips to heels

forehead toward the floor

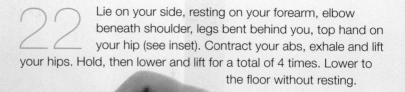

22 Lie on your side, resting on your forearm, elbow beneath shoulder, legs bent behind you, top hand on your hip (see inset). Contract your abs, exhale and lift your hips. Hold, then lower and lift for a total of 4 times. Lower to the floor without resting.

knees stacked, legs bent behind

feel it here

elbow is under the shoulder

23 Now add a "clam" to challenge your balance and stability. Open and close your top knee 4 times. Be sure to keep your rib cage lifted and the shoulder of your supporting arm down. Breathe naturally.

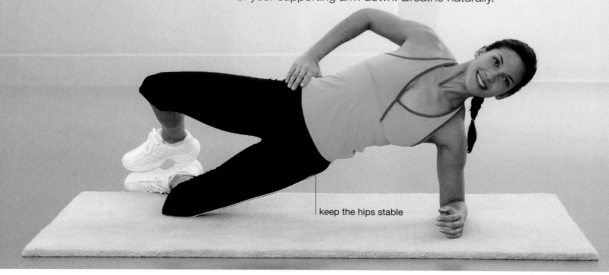

keep the hips stable

>> side stretch/wide "v" stretch

24 Lower your hips to the floor and sit up. Separating your legs, bend your knees to the side and reach your opposite arm overhead, palm down. Stretch out the muscles that you just worked, especially the obliques, and then repeat steps 22–24 on the other side.

keep the shoulder blade down

weight on the front hip

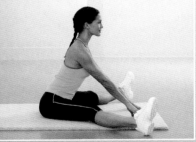

25 Sit tall and open your legs in a wide "V" (see inset). Lean forward from your hips with your spine straight, and reach your arms to center. Keeping both hips planted evenly on the floor, lift your spine, then turn your torso to face one leg, and hold. Pass through center and repeat on the other side.

spine straight

hips firmly planted

26 Bring your legs together, extended in front of you, torso facing forward. Bend one leg in, knee to ceiling, and cross it over the other, extended leg. Reach the arm on the same side as the bent knee behind you, hand on the floor (see inset), and twist your torso toward it, using the other arm on your knee to deepen the stretch. Hold, then switch sides.

use the opposite arm
on the bent knee

27 Turn your torso back to center. Straighten your spine, lift up and out of your lower back, and then reach your head forward. Relax over your knees, breathing deeply.

round over the legs

knees straight but not locked

core basics at a glance

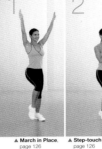
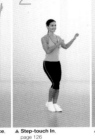
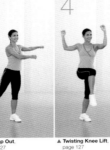
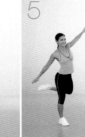
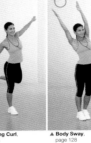

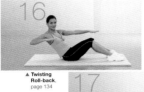

▲ Pelvic Tilt,
page 129

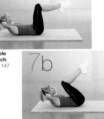

▲ March in Place,
page 126

▲ Step-touch In,
page 126

▲ Toe-tap Out,
page 127

▲ Twisting Knee Lift,
page 127

▲ Hamstring Curl,
page 128

▲ Body Sway,
page 128

▲ Straight-leg Lowering,
page 129

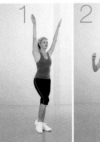

▲ Twisting
Roll-back,
page 134

▲ Kneeling Lift,
page 135

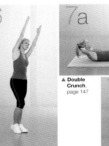

▲ Forearm Plank Plus,
page 136

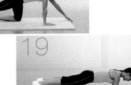

▲ Lengthening Stretch, page 134

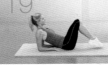

▲ Forearm Plank, page 135

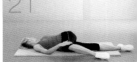

▲ Child's Pose, page 136

core challenge at a glance

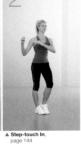
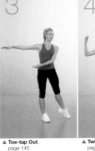

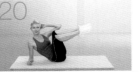

▲ Double
Crunch,
page 147

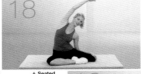

▲ Double Crunch, page 147

▲ March in Place,
page 144

▲ Step-touch In,
page 144

▲ Toe-tap Out,
page 145

▲ Twisting Knee Lift,
page 145

▲ Hamstring Curl,
page 146

▲ Body Sway,
page 146

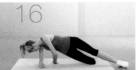

▲ Twisting Side
Plank,
page 152

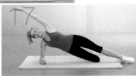

▲ Seated
Side
Stretch,
page 153

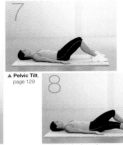

▲ Balance and
Crunch,
page 154

▲ Overhead Reach, page 152

▲ Toe Dip, page 153

▲ Crossover Stretch, page 154

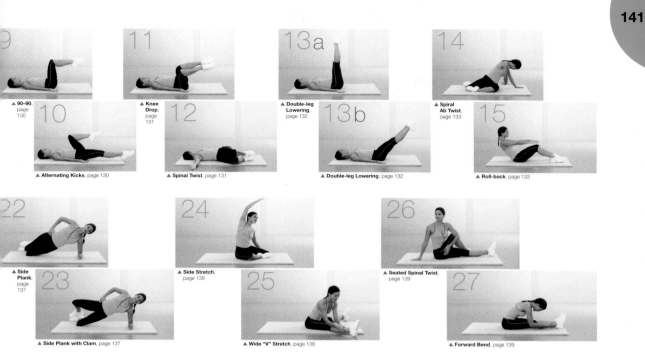

▲ **90–90**, page 130

▲ **Knee Drop**, page 131

▲ **Double-leg Lowering**, page 132

▲ **Spiral Ab Twist**, page 133

▲ **Alternating Kicks**, page 130

▲ **Spinal Twist**, page 131

▲ **Double-leg Lowering**, page 132

▲ **Roll-back**, page 133

▲ **Side Plank**, page 137

▲ **Side Stretch**, page 138

▲ **Seated Spinal Twist**, page 139

▲ **Side Plank with Clam**, page 137

▲ **Wide "V" Stretch**, page 138

▲ **Forward Bend**, page 139

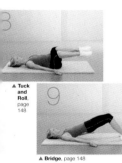

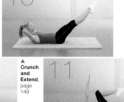

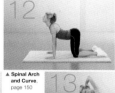

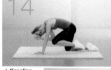

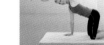

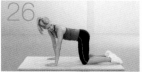

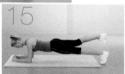

▲ **Tuck and Roll**, page 148

▲ **Crunch and Extend**, page 149

▲ **Spinal Arch and Curve**, page 150

▲ **Kneeling Crunch**, page 151

▲ **Bridge**, page 148

▲ **Dead Bug**, page 149

▲ **Kneeling Twist**, page 150

▲ **Plank with Leg Lift**, page 151

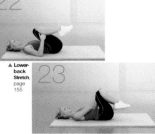

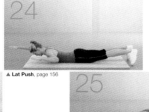

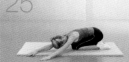

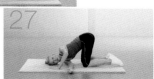

▲ **Lower-back Stretch**, page 155

▲ **Lat Push**, page 156

▲ **Alligator**, page 157

▲ **Circles**, page 155

▲ **Child's Pose**, page 156

▲ **Thread the Needle**, page 157

15 minute

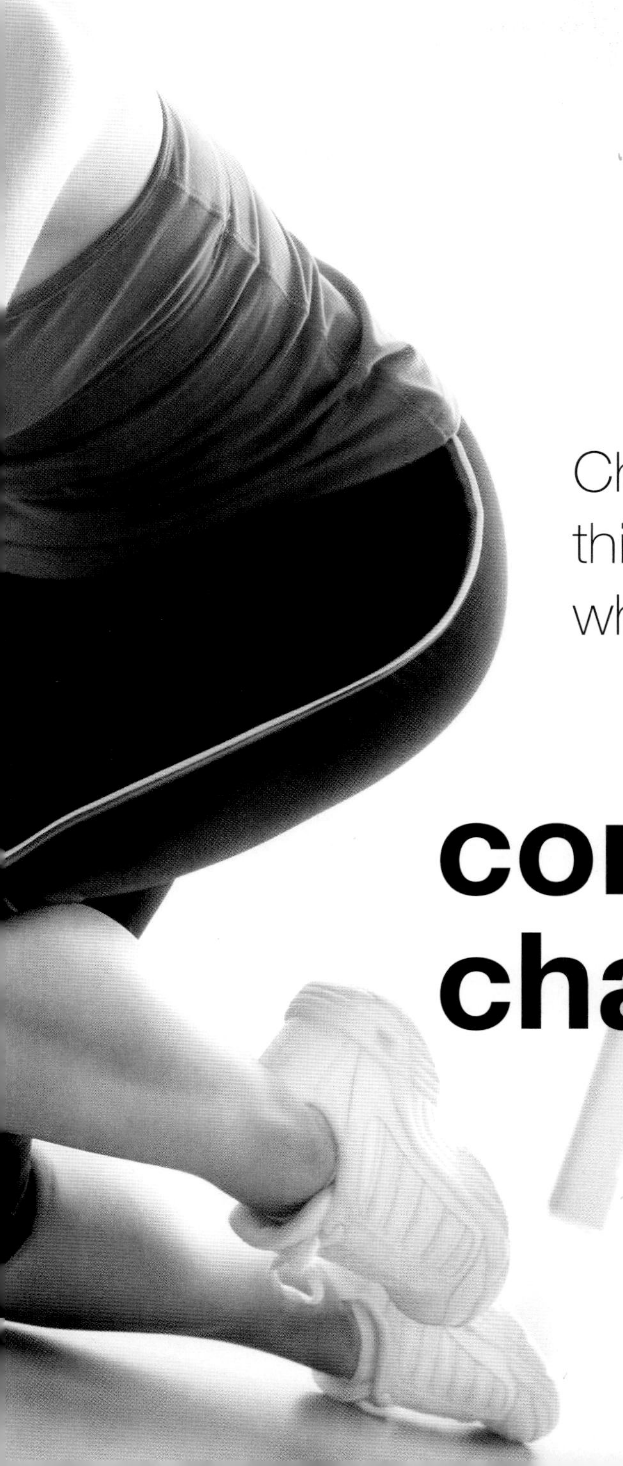

Challenge your core with
this more advanced routine
when you are ready

core
challenge >>

>> **march in place/step-touch in**

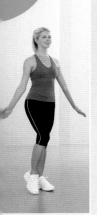

1 To warm up, begin marching with your feet parallel, knees soft, and arms by your sides (see inset). Add the arms, lifting them up with palms up, then down with palms down. March for 16 reps (1 rep = both sides).

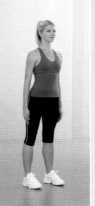

2 Step one leg to the side, arms by your sides (see inset). Step the other leg in, touching your feet together, bending your elbows to that side, and swinging your hands to shoulder height. Repeat, moving from side to side, for 8 reps.

turn the palms down as you lower the arms

keep the knee low

bend the elbows, fists to shoulder height

shift the weight from side to side

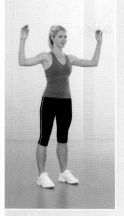

3 Step your feet apart, arms by your sides (see inset). Swing both arms to one side at shoulder height, coming up on the toes of the opposite foot. Circle your arms down to the other side and reach out with the tapping leg. Repeat, alternating sides for 8 reps.

4 With legs apart, raise the arms sideways to shoulder height. Bend your elbows to 90 degrees, palms forward (see inset). Keeping the back straight, bend one knee to hip height. Rotate your torso, bringing the opposite elbow toward the raised knee. Repeat, alternating sides for 8 reps.

arms swing like a pendulum

reach the tapping leg to the side

hold the torso upright

lift the knee to hip height

>> **hamstring curl/body sway**

5 Take your legs wider and reach your arms out to the sides at shoulder level, palms down (see inset). Bend one knee behind and reach for your foot with the opposite hand, raising the other arm up on a diagonal. Repeat, alternating sides for 8 reps.

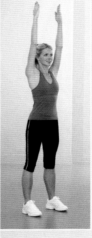

6 With legs apart and arms raised, step one leg in and flex at the waist (see inset). Keep your head centered between your arms. Repeat, alternating sides for 8 reps. **Repeat steps 5–1 (reverse order) to complete your warm up.**

stretch the
fingers

keep the shoulder
blades down

torso and head
move as one

reach the hand
to the foot

7a Raise one leg at a time to 90–90, knees above hips, calves parallel to the floor, and with a right angle at hips and knees (see p. 89). Place your unclasped hands behind your head. Exhale and lift the shoulder blades, keeping the abs tight.

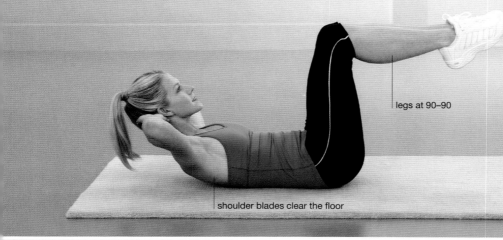

legs at 90–90

shoulder blades clear the floor

7b Hold the position as you curl your hips. Release the hips and then the shoulders, without resting your head on the floor. Repeat 10 times, then hug your knees to stretch your back.

right angle at knees

curl the hips off the floor

shoulders stay lifted

>> **tuck and roll/bridge**

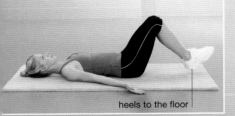

heels to the floor

8 Lying in 90–90, with legs together, arms by your sides and palms up, exhale, draw your abs in, then lower your legs and touch your heels lightly to the mat (see inset). Inhale, return to start, then exhale and roll your hips to the side, lowering your knees halfway. Inhale and return. Repeat the ab tuck, heels to the floor, then roll to the other side. Continue alternating sides for a total of 3 reps (1 rep = tuck/roll/tuck/roll).

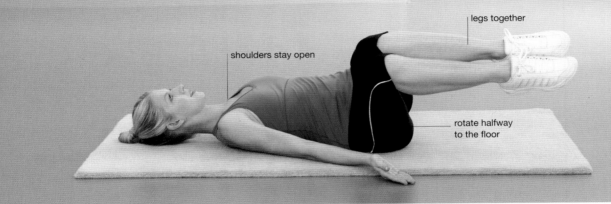

legs together

shoulders stay open

rotate halfway to the floor

9 Begin in neutral position, knees bent at 90 degrees, hip-width apart, feet flat, and arms by your sides, palms up (see inset). Inhale, then exhale, press your lower back to the floor, and begin lifting your hips, peeling your back off the floor until your hips form a straight line with your knees and shoulders. Inhale and release down one vertebra at a time. Repeat 3 times.

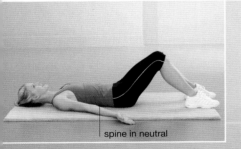

spine in neutral

maintain a neutral spine

90–90 position

10 Begin in 90–90, hands behind your head (see inset). Exhale, lift your chest to bring your shoulder blades off the floor at the same time as you extend your legs to 45 degrees, without arching your lower back. Inhale, and release back to start, keeping tension in your abs throughout. Repeat 5 times. Hug your knees to rest.

elbows wide

feel it here

legs at a 45 degree angle to the floor

11 Again, begin in 90–90, arms extended toward the ceiling, palms forward. Pull your abs tight, belly button to spine (see inset). Exhale and lower your opposite arm and leg toward the floor, bringing the other knee in over your chest. Switch sides for 6 reps, then add a hold for another 4 reps. Breathe naturally throughout. Hug your knees briefly.

bring the knee over the chest

lower without resting

feel it here

lower without resting

lower without resting

12 Kneel on all fours, wrists under shoulders, knees under hips, spine in neutral alignment. Exhale and round your back up to the ceiling, dropping your head between your arms and tucking your hips under (see inset). Inhale, lifting your head and hips, and curving your spine into a "C." Repeat twice each way.

wrists under the shoulders

knees under the hips

13 On all fours, stabilize one arm, spreading the fingers and pushing into the thumb and index finger to create a base of support. Place your other hand behind your head (see inset). Exhale and rotate your torso, elbow and head twisting as one. Inhale and return to start. Repeat 6 times.

keep the hips still

stabilize the arm

feel it here

press into the thumb and index finger

stabilize the supporting arm

14 Kneeling, one arm stabilized as in step 13, extend the other arm forward at shoulder level and the opposite leg back at hip height (see inset). Exhale, contract your abs, and round your back up to the ceiling as you draw elbow to knee, turning the palm up. Repeat 6 times, then switch sides and repeat steps 13 and 14.

rotate the arm, palm up

15 From a kneeling position, bend your elbows under your shoulders, hands in loose fists. Straighten one leg behind you, then the other. Contract the abs. Your body should form a straight line from shoulders to heels (see inset). Exhale and lift one leg, keeping the knee straight, then place that leg back down and lift the other. Continue for 6 reps, then sit back in Child's Pose (see p. 156).

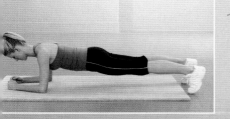

hands in loose fists

keep the hips level

core challenge >>

>> **twisting side plank/overhead reach**

look up at the hand

16 Lie on your side, hips stacked, bottom knee bent behind, top leg straight, and foot flexed. Plant your elbow under your shoulder, forearm on floor, hand in loose fist. Tighten your abs and lift your hips. Extend your top arm to the ceiling and look up at it (see inset). Exhale and twist, reaching your arm under your torso. Return to start and repeat for a total of 6 times.

feel it here

head follows the action

feel it here

17 Still in the side plank, reach your top arm overhead, palm down, stretching out the obliques while your core muscles work to maintain this position. Keep your head and neck aligned with your spine. Hold the stretch briefly.

hips stacked

abs tight

rib cage lifted

keep the shoulder blade down

weight on the front hip

18 Lower your hips from the side plank and come into a seated position with one leg bent behind and the other bent in front. Reach the arm on the same side as the front leg overhead toward the back knee, palm down. Hold for a moment, then swing your legs around to the other side to repeat steps 16–18.

19 Sit tall, both knees bent in front, feet flat. Lean back onto your elbows, shoulder blades down and together. Tighten your abs and slide your hands under your lower back for support, palms down. Lift your legs to 90–90 (see inset). Inhale and dip your toes to the mat, maintaining the right angle at the knees. Exhale, and return to start. Repeat 5 times.

anchor the shoulder blades

tap the toes lightly

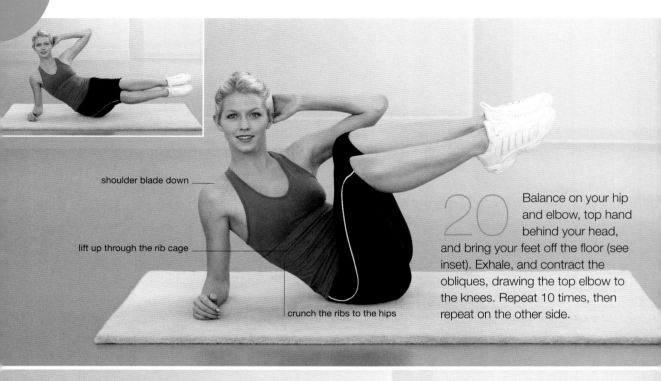

shoulder blade down

lift up through the rib cage

crunch the ribs to the hips

20 Balance on your hip and elbow, top hand behind your head, and bring your feet off the floor (see inset). Exhale, and contract the obliques, drawing the top elbow to the knees. Repeat 10 times, then repeat on the other side.

21 Stretch out on your back. Bend one knee up and use the opposite hand to guide it across your body into a Spinal Twist. Turn your head away from the bent knee. Rest the other arm to the side, palm up. Relax into the stretch, then change sides.

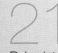

use the hand to deepen the stretch

22 Still lying on your back, return to center. Bend both knees up to your chest, separate them, and place your hands under your thighs. Inhale, then exhale as you pull your knees toward your shoulders, lifting your tailbone off the floor to gently stretch out your lower back.

draw the knees toward the shoulders

tailbone off the floor

23 Place your hands on top of your knees (see inset) and circle them together 3 times each way, massaging your lower back into the floor. Breathe naturally throughout and, with every exhale, think of releasing tension in your muscles.

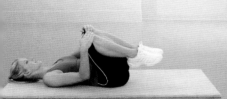

circle the knees together

>> lat push/child's pose

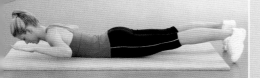

24 Turn onto your stomach, arms bent wide to the sides. Tuck your toes under, push onto the balls of your feet, knees off the floor. Scoop out your abs, draw your shoulders together in a "W," and lift your arms and head (see inset). Push one arm forward, then bring it back, alternating sides for a total of 5 reps.

draw the shoulder blades down and together

lift the knees off the floor

tuck the toes under

25 Sit back on your heels and bend forward, arms stretching out through your center. Keep your elbows off the mat to get the best stretch. Take deep breaths and relax into the position (see inset). Then, keeping your head centered between your elbows, walk your hands to one side and hold. Repeat to the other side.

keep the hips down

head between the elbows

elbows off the floor

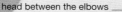

26 Come to a kneeling position, wrists under shoulders, knees under hips, spine in neutral alignment. Inhale, turn your head toward your hip. Exhale and return to center. Inhale to the other side; exhale and return. Continue moving side to side, using the breath to guide you for a total of 3 reps.

shoulders and hips move

27 This is a Spinal Twist from the knees. Starting on all fours, "thread" one arm under your body to the opposite side, palm up. Come to rest on your shoulder and the side of your head. Breathe into the stretch, feeling the elongation all along your side. Then change sides and thread the needle the other way.

rest on the shoulder and the side of head

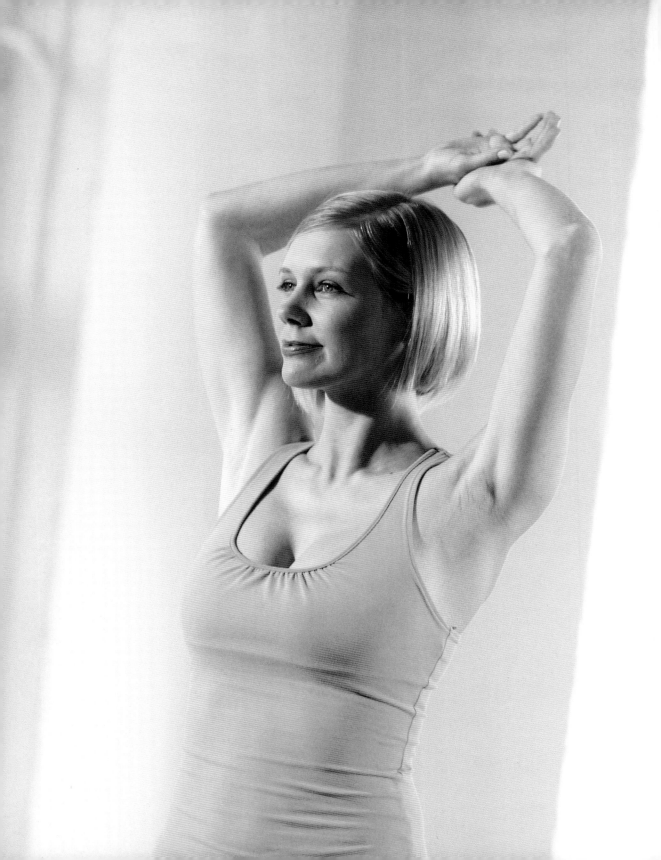

better back
workout

Suzanne Martin P.T., D.P.T.

>> **the parts of** the back

Take a moment at this point to review the four different parts of the back.

Each has a different role to play in enabling us to perform our everyday tasks.

Getting a clear idea of the four main sections of your back will help you

to make your exercises more effective. Look in the mirror and follow along.

The "back" is technically the "spine" and is made up of several parts. Looking from the side, it makes a long S-curve. The spine has four main curves: the cervical, the thoracic, the lumbar, and the fused sacral/coccyx. The curves are not present at birth and only begin to develop when an infant achieves vertical standing and at toddler stage when he or she begins to walk. The downward press of gravity shapes the spine and gives each curve an all-important role in maintaining the health of the back and producing bipedal stance.

The cervical spine

The cervical spine or upper neck can be felt at your hairline, just at the base of the skull. It is responsible for tipping the chin upward and downward. The upper part of the cervical spine also contains the muscles responsible for eye motions. If you keep your fingertips at the base and dart your eyes back and forth, you'll detect the motions of these fine muscles.

The lower cervical spine is convex-shaped. You can usually feel the prominent southernmost vertebra as it meets the shoulders. The neck has the greatest amount of range of motion of the spine. It can create a telescoping effect and can swivel to almost look completely behind you.

The thoracic spine

This has a concave shape and is connected with the rib cage. You can trace the prominent spinous processes, the visible bumps of the spine, by

> ## >> **the four main** parts of the back
>
> - **The cervical spine**, or "neck," has seven vertebrae and extends from the base of the skull to the shoulders.
> - **The thoracic spine**, comprising the upper and mid-back, has 12 vertebrae and extends from the shoulders to the waist.
> - **The lumbar spine**, or "lower back," has five vertebrae. This vulnerable section forms the waist and has no bony support.
> - **The sacral section** contains the four fused vertebrae of the sacrum with the vestigial tail, the "coccyx," at its end.

running your thumbs from your shoulders down to the top of your waist. It is chronically stiff since it's girdled by the rib cage, so developing mobility in the thoracic spine requires patience.

The lumbar spine

Put your hands around your waist to find the lumbar spine. This part of the spine is particularly vulnerable because it's balancing the weight of the trunk against the unwieldy weighty legs. What's special about the lumbar spine is its springboard effect on the spine. Its convex shape allows the impact against the ground to dissipate as you step.

The back is not a single entity but is actually made up of four main sections. The exercises in *Better Back Workout* will help you strengthen each of them.

The curves make an S-shape that gives the back resilience. Preserving those curves is all-important if you want a pain-free back!

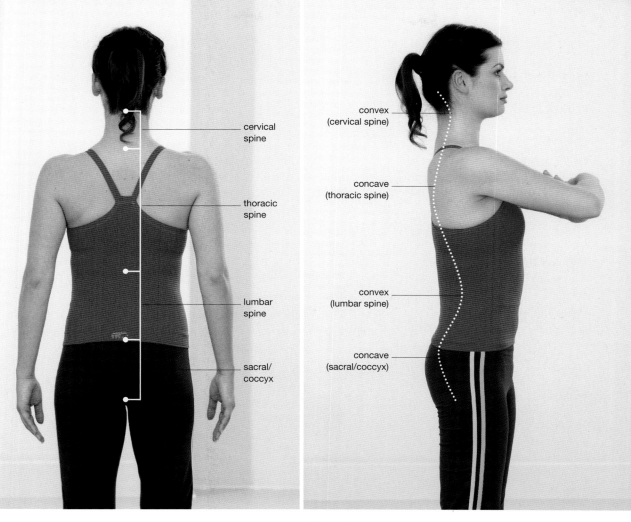

cervical spine

thoracic spine

lumbar spine

sacral/ coccyx

convex (cervical spine)

concave (thoracic spine)

convex (lumbar spine)

concave (sacral/coccyx)

The sacrum

Finally, place your hands on your hip bones, fingers facing forward, and your thumbs will end up on top of the fused vertebrae of the sacrum. Very large forces converge here—at the sacroiliac joints—the place where the lumbar spine and the sacrum meet. That means that this area is extremely vulnerable and requires careful positioning and handling if you are to avoid injury. At the bottom of this fusion lies the coccyx or tailbone.

The discs

These are pieces of cartilage that lie between the vertebrae. Think of them as being like jelly donuts, with a soft center and a hard exterior. They provide cushioning in between the vertebrae but, even more importantly, they give range to the spine so it can bend and twist as required. Protecting the spine means protecting these all-important discs. And that is achieved by strengthening the back and by learning posture control.

>> **posture** and the back

Posture is important both to the strength of your back and to how you appear. It can make you look dumpy, tired, and old, or together, confident, and lithe. Fortunately, posture is not all down to your genetic inheritance. There is much you can do to improve it and prevent gravity from winning out.

The slump

This posture pushes the head forward out of line, rounds the shoulders, and leads to a slouched pelvis. Besides being esthetically unappealing, it places enormous strain on the discs.

The sway back

Runway models perform the sway to make themselves appear "cool." The sway back posture makes the shoulders lean and compresses the lower spine while reversing the thoracic area. In a nutshell—stand up straight!

Hyperlordosis

This is an exaggerated curve of the lumbar spine. It weakens the springboard effect provided by the lower back to the rest of the spine. It also shortens the stabilizing muscles of the pelvis. It's not only pregnant women and those with apple-body types who fall into this category. Athletic people tend to get tight hips that can throw them into this posture.

Below left to right The slump, the sway back, and hyperlordosis are three typical bad postures. Each will cause problems for the body sooner or later.

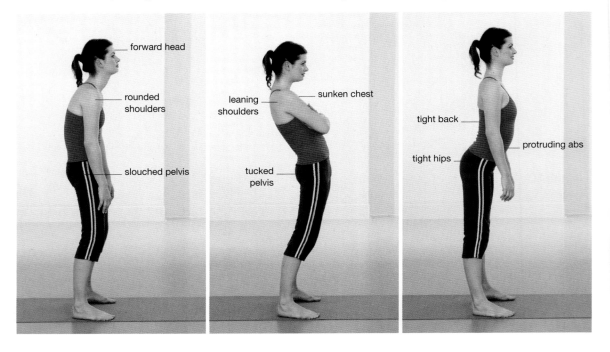

forward head

rounded shoulders

slouched pelvis

leaning shoulders

sunken chest

tucked pelvis

tight back

tight hips

protruding abs

See the difference between bad and good posture. On the left, bad posture is sure to mean aches and pains. On the right, good posture looks healthy and is healthy.

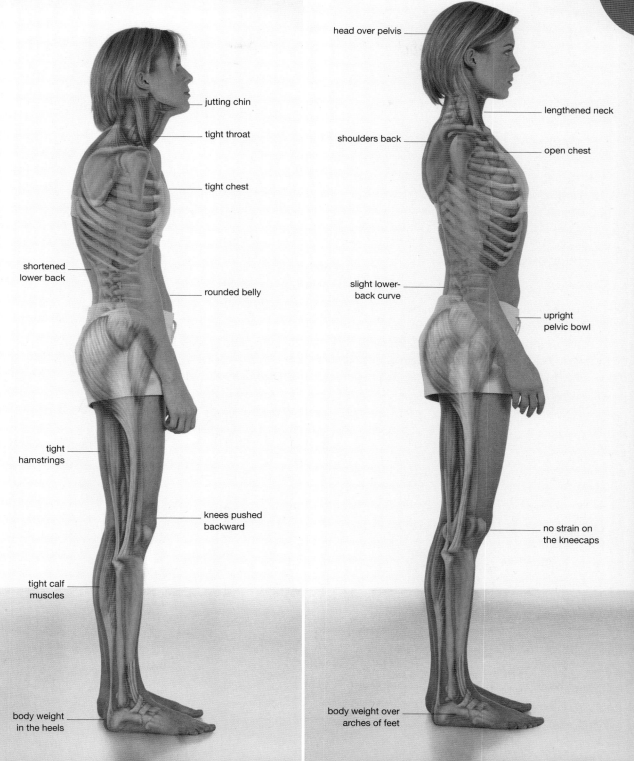

jutting chin

tight throat

tight chest

shortened lower back

rounded belly

tight hamstrings

knees pushed backward

tight calf muscles

body weight in the heels

head over pelvis

lengthened neck

shoulders back

open chest

slight lower-back curve

upright pelvic bowl

no strain on the kneecaps

body weight over arches of feet

>> **protecting** the back

The back requires extra protection because it has so many interconnecting parts. If one part gets injured, so do all the others. There are certain moves we all perform every day that involve the back. Performing them correctly, as shown here, can go a long way in protecting the spine.

First position parallel means bringing your feet straight under your pelvis. It is the healthiest position to adopt for the legs and gives the greatest support for the spine.

"Butt-ski, out-ski" is the humorous name for this bending position (below right). It is ergonomically best for the discs of the lower back, which can be severely and irreparably damaged when bending, and particularly when lifting and twisting at the same time. It's really simple; just think of bending from the hips, sticking the bottom out, and using the legs to take the strain as you stand up.

The log roll is particularly helpful, especially for getting in and out of bed or up and down from lying on the floor. It's an excellent strategy when your back is painful and sore. It's shown on the opposite page in four simple steps.

Below left For first position parallel take the feet about 4 inches (10 cm) apart, with the second toe lining up with the kneecap and with the point midway on the groin line.

Below When you are bending, bend at the hips and keep the back straight. For lifting, always think "butt-ski, out-ski" (stick the bottom out) and lift with the legs.

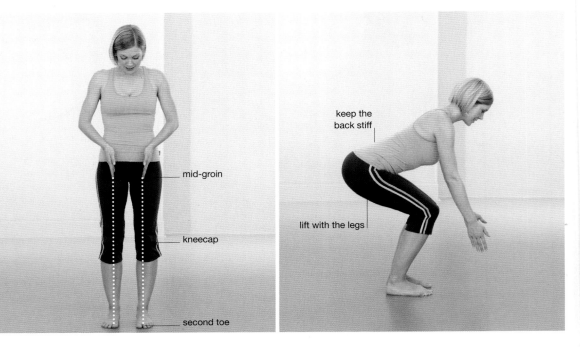

mid-groin

kneecap

second toe

keep the back stiff

lift with the legs

log roll to get up safely

1 First, while lying on your back, tighten your waist and abdomen. Next, keep your back stiff just as in the "butt-ski, out-ski" position (see opposite) and brace your bent legs.

2 Roll onto your side as a unit with your shoulders and hips; don't twist at your waist. Keep your legs together. When getting out of bed, let your feet go over the side.

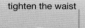

tighten the waist

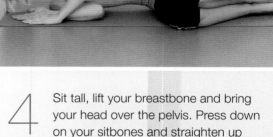

keep the waist stiff

3 Next, use your arms, not your back, to push yourself up to sitting. When getting out of bed, let your feet dangle over the edge as soon as possible.

4 Sit tall, lift your breastbone and bring your head over the pelvis. Press down on your sitbones and straighten up through your spine. Feel as if your spine is being sucked up through a straw toward your head.

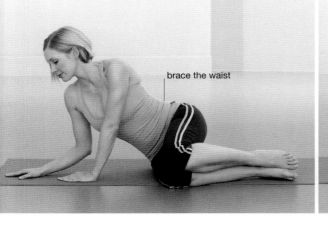

brace the waist

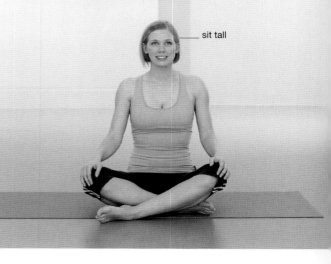

sit tall

>> **imagery** and cues

I like to use imagery and cues when I teach. They make all the difference to how you execute the movements and so will help you gain maximum benefit from the exercises. Here are some of the images demystified for you. Get to know them to bring more quality and greater detail to your movements.

The imagery I use is for you to hold in your mind when you are making a movement, just as an actor imagines and acts out a role during a performance. It is the same when someone is exercising. The phrases, or cues, guide the exerciser to know exactly how and when to execute the movement. You will quickly become familiar with the imagery and cues and you'll find that they promote the concentration and complexity needed to make your exercise more precise, and so most effective.

Follow the cues

Make smile lines These are two arc shapes that can be seen at the very tops of the legs when you tighten the hips and the backs of the thighs. They mark the separation of the muscles of the buttocks and the hamstrings.

Go into tabletop position is an image used to help you get your entire back, when you are on all fours, parallel to the floor. Your back should look just like the flat surface of a tabletop.

Imagine pressing pearls into sand is a term used to help you articulate each individual vertebra of the

Below left "Smile lines" delineate the buttocks from the hamstrings. **Center** "Pull the navel to the spine" tells you to bring the abs in firmly. **Below right** "Zip up the tight jeans" helps you to lift the abs.

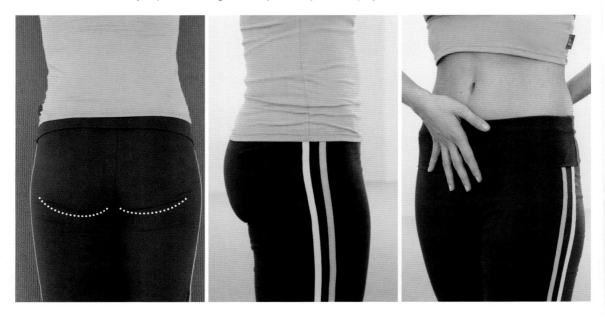

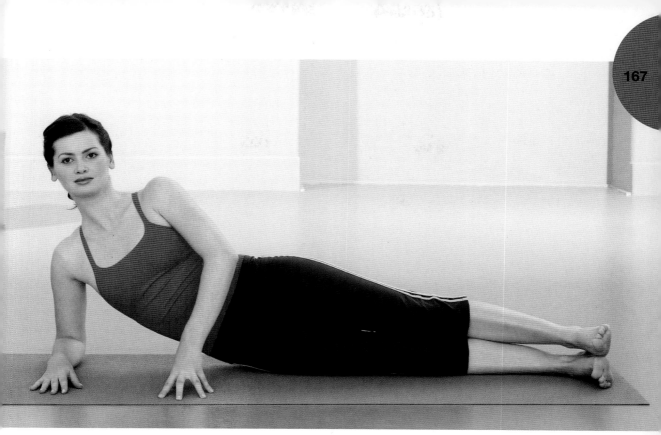

Above In this exercise, one of the keys to achieving a good pose is to feel the navel engaging to the spine—in other words, pulling the abdominal muscles firmly inward.

spine separately. When you are lying on your back, after lifting your pelvis off the floor, you lower the spine sequentially, one vertebra at a time, imagining as you do so that each vertebra is pressing a pearl, or bead, into soft sand beneath your body.

Take the head over the pelvis helps to ensure correct posture by eliminating slumping and a forward head.

Feel imaginary hands creating a sandwiching effect helps you to coordinate abdominal tension with back tension to give a stiffer, straighter trunk.

Imagine swimming pool water is used when your abdomen is facing the floor to make you feel as if water is pressing upward against your abdomen. It helps you to lift the contents of your abdomen.

Lift the pelvis means to engage the muscles that stop the flow of urine and that stop you from breaking wind. Gently feel these muscles pull up toward your head, just as you would lift the arches of your feet to keep your ankles from wobbling.

Funnel the ribs helps you achieve a better upper-body crunch. First you "deflate" the breastbone, meaning that you compress it toward the ground. Then, as you start to curl your shoulders off the floor, you literally pull your ribs toward your pelvis, instead of just hinging at the waist.

Pull the navel to the spine means to pull the abdominals strongly inward.

Zip up the tight jeans means to lift the abdominals upward from the pubic bone toward the navel. It is the movement you need to zip up tight jeans.

Go into puppy dog position means lying on your back with your legs and arms bent and off the floor. This allows you to engage your core muscles fully.

Imagine a dog's tail between the legs gives precision when you are doing pelvic tilts lying on your back. The image helps you curl your pelvis into a rounded shape as you imagine the connection between the fused vertebrae of your sacrum and the coccyx or very end of your spine.

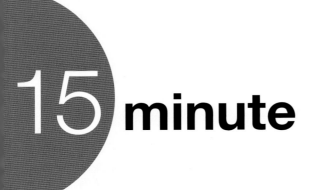

15 minute

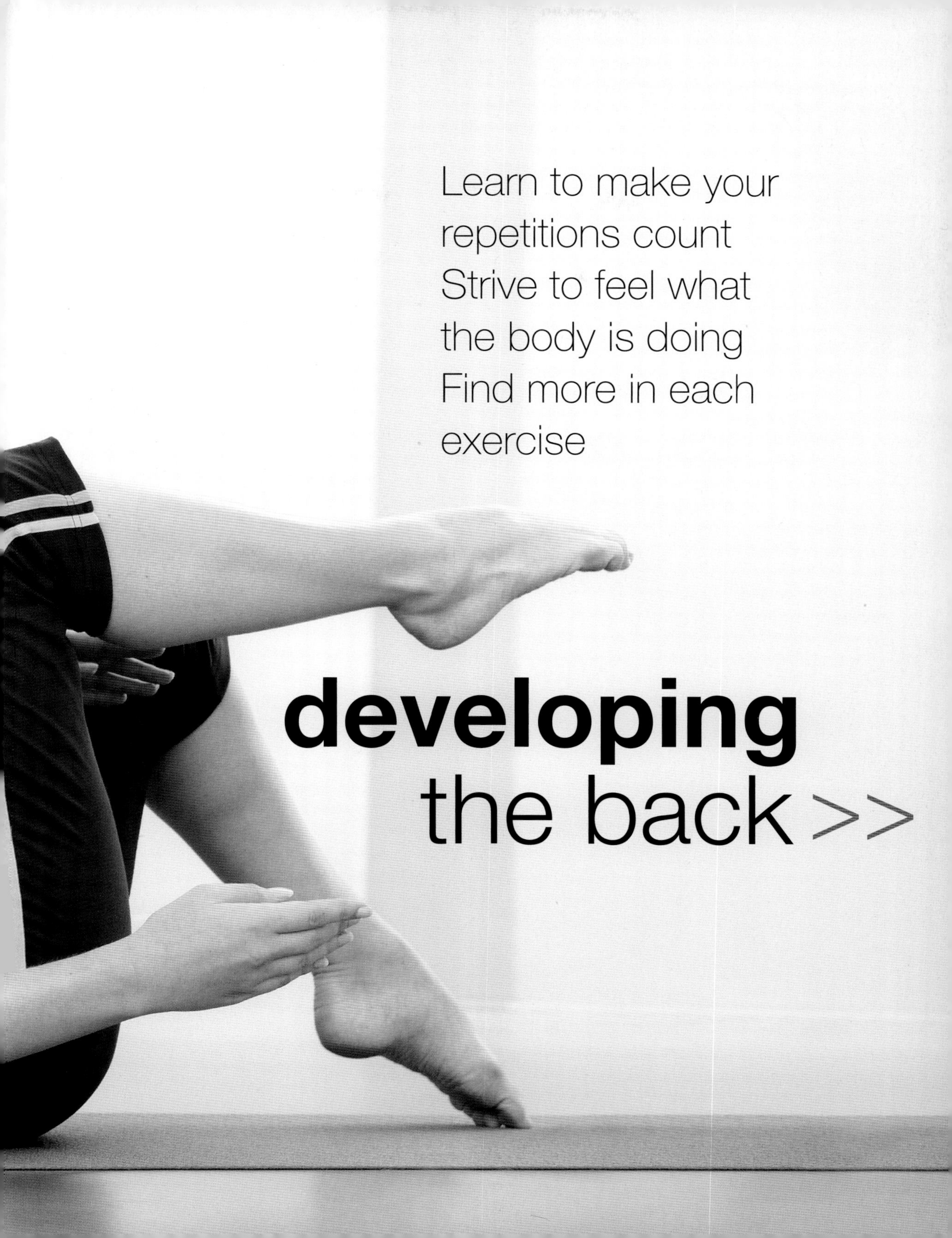

Learn to make your
repetitions count
Strive to feel what
the body is doing
Find more in each
exercise

developing
the back >>

>> **upper rolls**

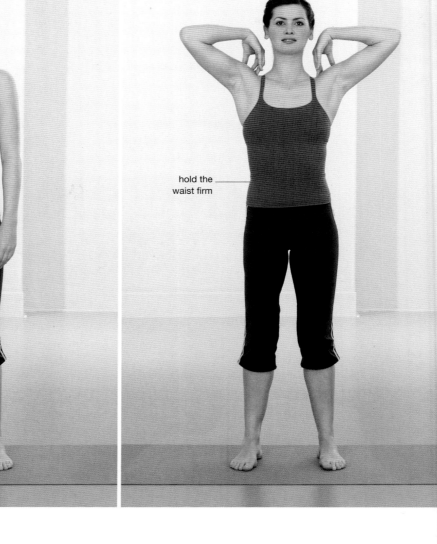

1 Stand tall with your feet about shoulder-width apart (see inset). Zip up the tight jeans (see p. 167) in the front and in the back. Open your chest and take your head over your pelvis (see p. 167). Breathe in and out as you count to 8 while slowly rolling your shoulders backward.

2 Hold your waist firm. Fold your elbows, and bring your hands to your shoulders. Make full, yet comfortable circles with your elbows about 5 times. Then reverse the direction for 5 more circles.

roll the
shoulders
backward

hold the
waist firm

>> **body yawn**

3 Place your feet just past shoulder-width apart (see inset). Reach your arms up sideways with your palms facing forward. Reach up and wide. Open your mouth and eyes.

reach up
strongly

4 Balance on your left leg, then exhale and squeeze your right knee to your waist. Find your balance, then return to stand on both feet with your arms reaching upward. Now balance on your right leg and squeeze your left knee to your waist. Repeat this alternation from right to left for 3 more sets.

keep the
hip firm

take the feet just
past shoulder width

developing the back >>

>> **knee circles**

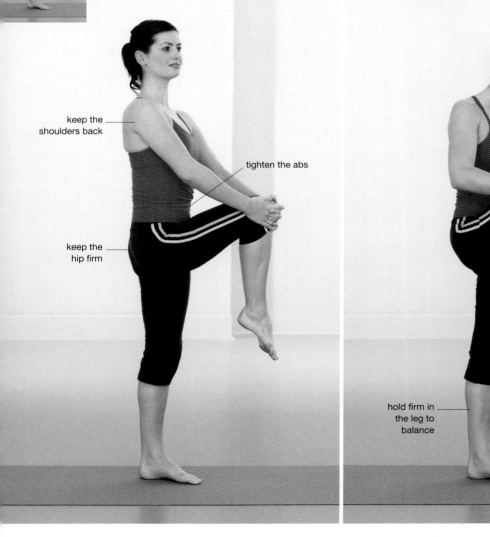

5 Stand on your left leg and be aware of your balance. Tighten your abs and hold your right knee steady to your waist with both hands (see inset). Anchor your shoulders back. Hold onto a piece of furniture if you can't manage to balance. Circle your knee 3 times.

6 Exhale and bow your head to your right knee and feel the stretch in your back. Release. Stand on your right leg and repeat the balance and circles. End with a bow to your left knee.

keep the shoulders back

tighten the abs

keep the hip firm

hold firm in the leg to balance

7 Stand and balance on your right leg. Cross your left foot over in front of your right ankle (see inset). Reach your right arm up and over your head toward the left.

reach up through the fingers

8 Zip up the tight jeans and firmly push your left hand in a horizontal motion against your left hip so you bend to the left. Breathe in and out 4 times. Come back to center. Uncross your leg and repeat to stretch your left side the same way.

feel it here

hold the abs

tuck the hip in

>> **squat stretch**

9 Open your legs past shoulder width and turn your toes slightly outward (see inset). Hold your waist tight and firm your bottom as you bend straight down inside your legs to place your hands on top of your knees.

10 Lift your pelvis (see p. 167) and lengthen your spine. Inhale, press your right hand against your right knee, then exhale and turn your shoulders to look diagonally up and to your left. Breathe in and out 3 times. Stand up, then repeat the stretch to the other side.

press down on the thighs for support

check that the toes are visible

feel it here

feel it here

lift the pelvic muscles toward the head

>> toe touches

11 Lie down with your knees bent. Exhale, curl up your upper body, reach your hands out past your thighs, and take your feet off the floor (see inset). Look along your body. Take your left arm between your legs, reaching ahead with your middle fingers, and pull your head to your groin. Now lightly touch the toes of your left foot to the floor.

press the lower back into the floor

strongly reach the middle fingers out parallel to the floor

12 Simultaneously touch the right foot to the floor as you raise the left. Alternate toe touches for 16 repetitions. Place your right arm between your legs and alternate toe touches 16 more times. To end, hold both legs and arms up and increase the pull of your middle fingers.

intensify by reaching harder with the fingers

>> side bends

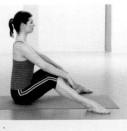

13 Sit on your sitbones with your legs shoulder-width apart and the soles of your feet on the floor (see inset). If you can't sit up straight, sit on a book or pillow. Line your head up directly over your pelvis. Place your hands behind your head and feel the "V" of strength running in a line from your lower back up and out of your elbows. Take your navel to your spine (see p. 167).

lift the skin of the
lower back upward

place the soles of
the feet on the floor

14 Lift up and over an imaginary fence with your right ribs as you reach your right elbow toward your right knee. Feel your left elbow point up toward the ceiling. Exhale and press down on your right sitbone to lift up to return to the "V" position of strength. Repeat to the left and then once more to each side.

reach up with
the top elbow

feel it here

keep the ribs lifted
on the lower side—
don't collapse

>> **overhead squeeze**

sit tall

turn the palms upward

keep the lower
back lifted

15 Sit with your legs crossed and your middle fingers out to the sides on the floor (see inset). Exhale and float your hands up sideways. At shoulder height, turn your palms upward.

cross the thumbs
and press the little
fingers together

stay lifted

16 Continue reaching upward until your hands meet over your head. Cross your thumbs, press your palms together, and squeeze your upper arms against your head. Then exhale, sit taller, and open your arms back down. Keep your spine tall as you lower your arms sideways, turning your palms downward as you reach shoulder-height. Take your middle fingers to the floor. Repeat once more.

>> **temple**

17 Lie on your front. Feel the imaginary swimming pool water lift your abs off the floor (see p. 167). Reach your hands above your head on the floor, with elbows bent and palms together (see inset). Knit your ribs together to engage your solar plexus. Tuck your toes under to make little stands. Make smile lines (see p. 166).

pull the tailbone
toward the heels

tuck the toes under

18 Inhale, then exhale as you levitate your hands and forearms off the floor, while at the same time straightening your knees so they come off the floor as well. Stay as you take a couple of breaths, then exhale and lower. Relax and then repeat the sequence.

anchor the hips

lift the abs

>> oppositional lifts

19 Go onto all fours. Feel the swimming pool water underneath your torso. Keep your elbows a little bent (see inset). Exhale and slide your second toe of your right foot behind you until your knee is straight, and at the same time slide your left middle finger out along the floor until your elbow is straight.

toe barely touches
the floor

fingers
barely
touch the
floor

20 Exhale and levitate your right foot and left hand up until they are horizontal. Stay and inhale, then exhale as you lower just to touch your fingertip and tops of your toes to the floor. Reach out and away from your torso to repeat. Breathe and lower. Repeat to the other side.

feel it here

avoid any swing
of the hip

feel it here

feel it here

>> plank push-up

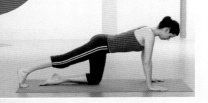

21

Go onto all fours. Feel the imaginary swimming pool water up against your abs and hands sandwiching your lower back (see p. 167). Exhale and reach your right leg behind you and tuck your toes under to make a stand (see inset). Then exhale and reach the left leg behind you. This position is called a full Plank.

tuck the toes under

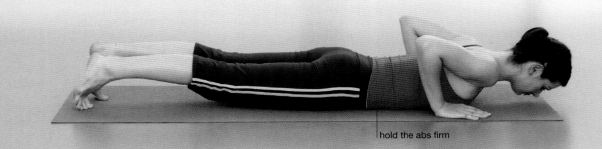

22

Inhale, bend your elbows, and lower yourself in push-up style. Make smile lines. Exhale and stay, then inhale, exhale, and come back up. Feel as if your abs have lifted you. Break at one hip and then the other to return to all fours. Repeat once more.

hold the abs firm

>> **angel wings**

23 Lie on your back. Feel the breath filling your torso as you inhale. Stretch your ankles away from your head. Lengthen your body (see inset). Exhale, then make angel wings with your arms, sliding your hands toward your hips as you bend your knees, raise your feet, and drag your feet toward your hips.

take the feet toward the hips

make angel wings with the arms

24 Reach to grab your heels, curling your body up into a little ball. Then inhale, lengthen your hips and legs down onto the floor again, and repeat 3 more times. Hold and intensify the last curl, tightening your abs, then relax to the floor.

curl up into a ball

developing the back at a glance

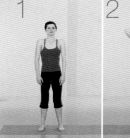

1

▲ Upper Rolls, page 170

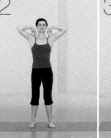

2

▲ Upper Rolls, page 170

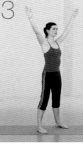

3

▲ Body Yawn, page 171

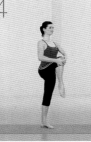

4

▲ Body Yawn, page 171

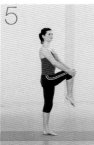

5

▲ Knee Circles, page 172

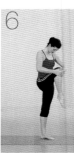

6

▲ Knee Circles, page 172

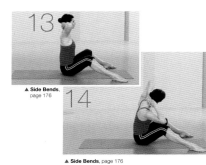

13

▲ Side Bends, page 176

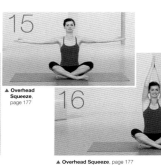

15

▲ Overhead Squeeze, page 177

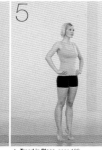

17

▲ Temple, page 178

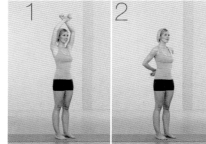

14

▲ Side Bends, page 176

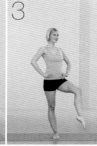

16

▲ Overhead Squeeze, page 177

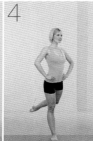

18

▲ Temple, page 178

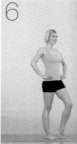

revitalizing the back at a glance

1

▲ Arm Swing, page 186

2

▲ Arm Swing, page 186

3

▲ Leg Swing, page 187

4

▲ Leg Swing, page 187

5

▲ Tread in Place, page 188

6

▲ Tread in Place, page 188

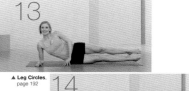

13

▲ Leg Circles, page 192

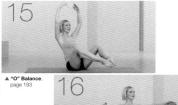

15

▲ "O" Balance, page 193

17

▲ Prone Rocker, page 194

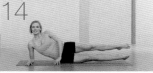

14

▲ Leg Circles, page 192

16

▲ "O" Balance, page 193

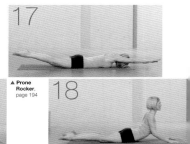

18

▲ Prone Rocker, page 194

7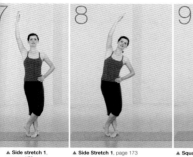
▲ Side stretch 1, page 173

8
▲ Side Stretch 1, page 173

9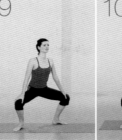
▲ Squat Stretch, page 174

10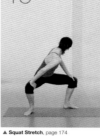
▲ Squat Stretch, page 174

11
▲ Toe Touches, page 175

12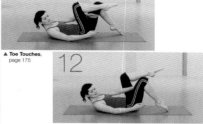
▲ Toe Touches, page 175

19
▲ Oppositional Lifts, page 179

20
▲ Oppositional Lifts, page 179

21
▲ Plank Push-up, page 180

22
▲ Plank Push-up, page 180

23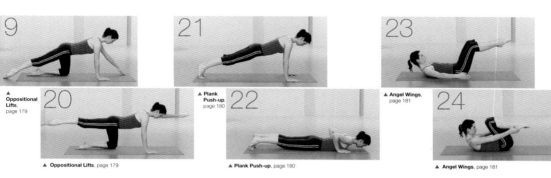
▲ Angel Wings, page 181

24
▲ Angel Wings, page 181

7
▲ Tapping Chest, page 189

8
▲ Tapping Chest, page 189

9
▲ Side Stretch 2, page 190

10
▲ Side Stretch 2, page 190

11
▲ Stroke the Cat, page 191

12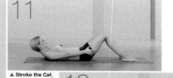
▲ Stroke the Cat, page 191

19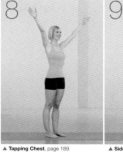
▲ Rest Breather, page 195

20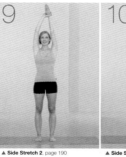
▲ Rest Breather, page 195

21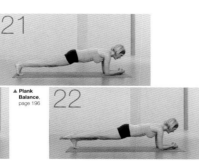
▲ Plank Balance, page 196

22
▲ Plank Balance, page 196

23
▲ "C" Exercise, page 197

24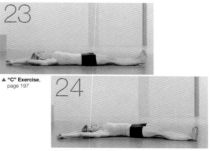
▲ "C" Exercise, page 197

15 minute

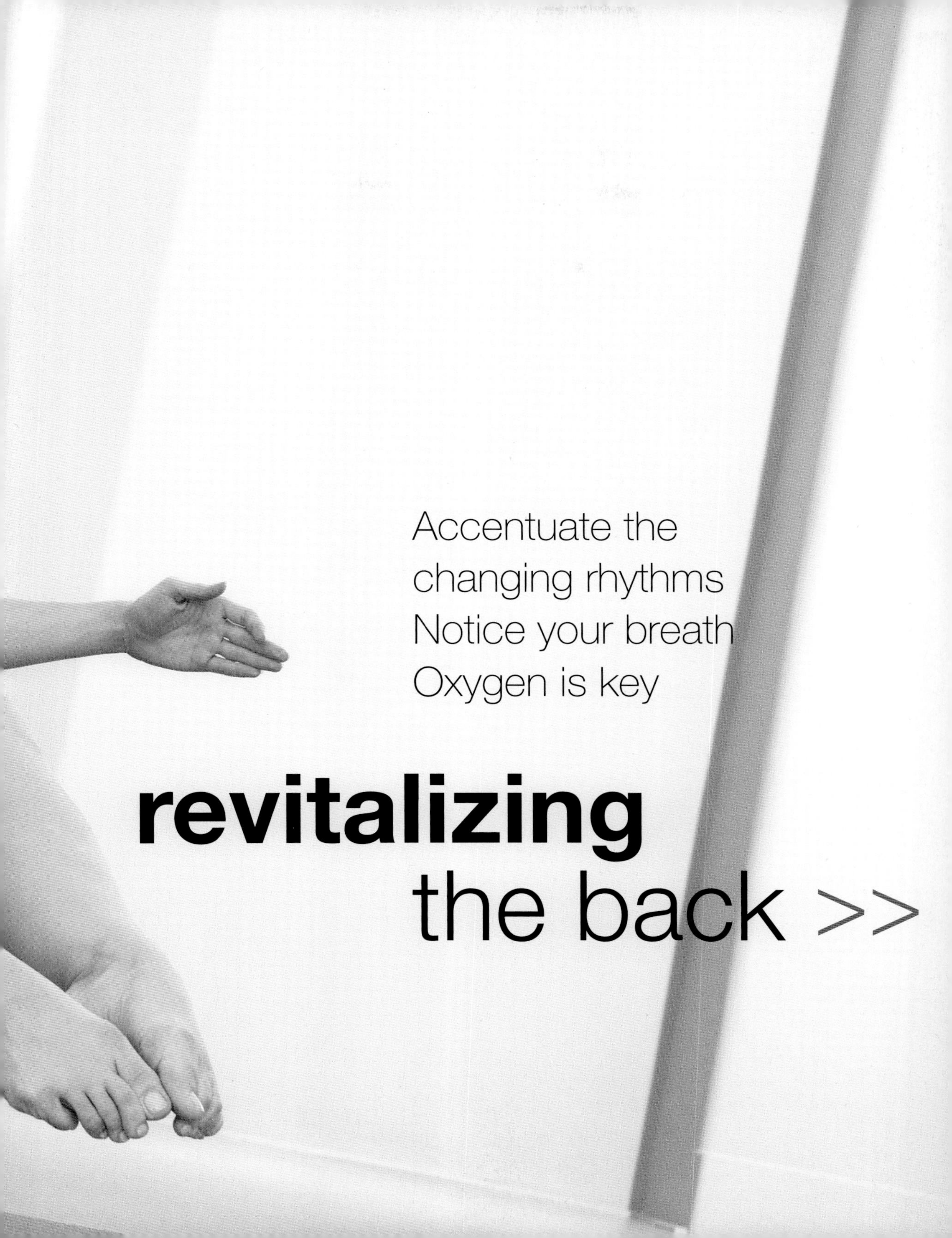

Accentuate the
changing rhythms
Notice your breath
Oxygen is key

revitalizing
the back >>

>> arm swing

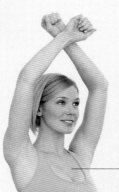

1 Place your feet just past shoulder-width apart with your toes turned slightly outward. Zip up the tight jeans (see p. 167). Ground your feet. Cross your wrists in front of you (see inset), then swing them up to your head with your palms facing outward.

2 Swing your hands back and behind your hips so they touch together. Rhythmically swing your arms up and back using this motion 7 more times.

keep the chest up

lengthen the waist

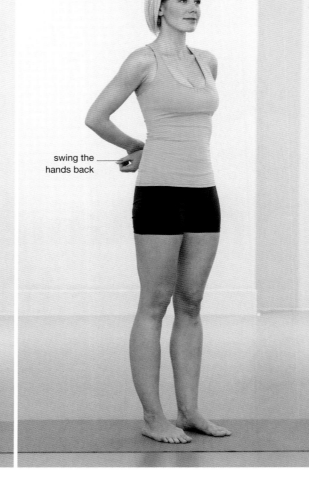

swing the hands back

3 Stand tall with your hands on your hips (see inset). Balance on your right leg, using a hand on a piece of furniture to support you if you need. Hold your hip firm on your right leg. Keep your chest up. Swing your left foot in front, as if you were wiping your foot on the ground.

4 Then swing your left foot down and back. Repeat this forward and backward motion easily and rhythmically 7 more times. Find your balance on your left leg and repeat, swinging your right leg.

hold the hip firm on the balance leg

swing the leg rhythmically

>> tread in place

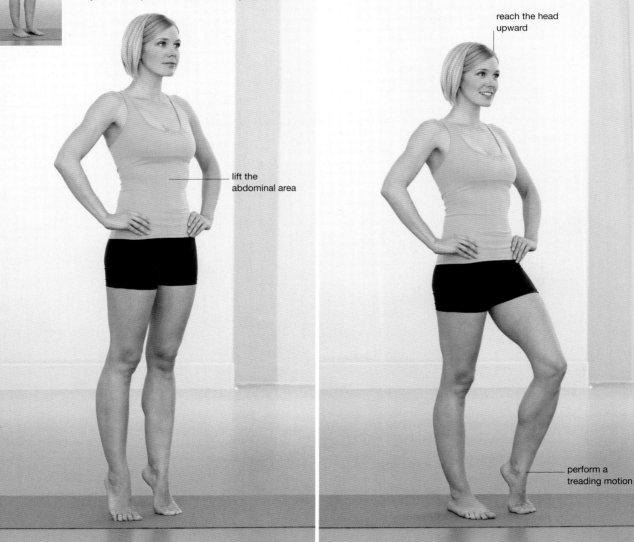

5 Stand tall with your feet just less than hip-width apart, hands on your hips (see inset). Take your head back over your pelvis and pull your navel to your spine (see p. 167). Lift your abdominal area from your pubis to your navel. Let this lift help you rise up onto the balls of your feet.

6 Reach your head upward as you lower your right heel, then rise up on the balls of your feet and lower your left heel. Repeat this treading motion 32 times.

lift the
abdominal area

reach the head
upward

perform a
treading motion

>> **tapping chest**

7 Stand tall with your feet just less than hip-width apart. Take your head back over your pelvis, pull your navel to your spine, lift your abs. Bring both hands to your breastbone (see inset). Gently tap your fingers on your breastbone as you exhale, saying "ha, ha, ha, ha" as you tap.

8 Now inhale as you open your arms, making two big rainbow shapes up and out to the sides. Take your hands back to your breastbone and repeat the motion 4 more times, alternating the exhalation "ha"s with the inhalation rainbow shapes.

exhale as you tap the chest

lift the abs

feel it here

feel it here

feel it here

>> side stretch 2

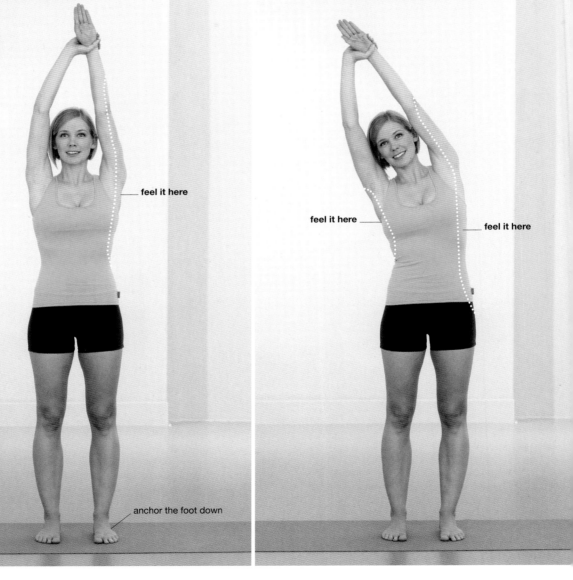

9 Stand with your arms above your head, and your feet about hip-width apart (see inset). Anchor your left foot downward as you grasp your left wrist with your right hand. Elongate and pull your wrist upward.

10 Inhale as you lift up, to the right, as though you were leaning over a fence. Stay, exhale, lengthen. Then inhale, stay, then exhale and anchor your left foot again as you stretch back up to vertical, lengthening your waistline. Take your arms down. Repeat to the other side.

feel it here

feel it here

feel it here

anchor the foot down

>> **stroke the cat**

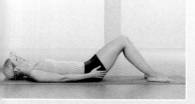

11 Lie on your back and bend your knees. Open your feet about shoulder-width apart. Place your left hand behind your head and hold behind your right thigh with your right hand (see inset). Exhale, deflate your breastbone, and funnel your ribs (see p. 167) toward your pelvis to curl up your upper body. Use your left arm to pull up higher.

hold the abs
firmly in

press the lower back
against the floor

12 Now stroke your right thigh from bottom to top with your right hand, as if you were stroking a cat. Reach out past your knee with your middle finger. Stroke 6 times, then intensify the last stroke. Lower your upper body to the floor, then change arms to repeat, using your left hand and stroking your left thigh 6 times.

reach past the knee
with the middle finger

>> leg circles

13 Lie on your right side in a straight line. Prop yourself up on your right forearm, using your left hand for balance (see inset). If you can't do this, lie on your shoulder with your arm folded and your hand around your neck to make a "pillow." Exhale and levitate your legs off the floor, then rotate them to create a "V" shape with your feet.

push the hips forward

take the heels together, toes apart

keep the waistline and ribs lifted

14 Now make tiny circles with your left leg, leading with your second toe. Do 2 sets of 10 repetitions circling in one direction. Then reverse and do 2 sets of 10 repetitions in the opposite direction. Roll to the other side and repeat, then lower your legs and relax.

feel it here

feel it here

>> "O" balance

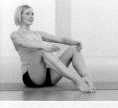

15 Sit and balance on your sitbones. Bend your legs and bring your ankles toward your hips. Make a circle around your knees with your arms (see inset). Exhale and draw your shoulder blades down. Inhale, exhale again, then lift your feet off the ground to balance on your sitbones as you move your arms to an "O" shape.

balance on the sitbones

16 Stay, feeling yourself getting taller, then exhale, press your hips down to the floor, open your arms, and take your arms back down to your knees. Repeat 2 more times.

lift the lower back

>> **prone rocker**

17 Lie on the front of your body. Reach your hands above your head on the floor about shoulder-width apart, palms face down. Exhale and drag your hands toward your upper chest to make the sphinx pose (see inset). Exhale, and levitate your feet off the floor about 2 inches (5 cm). Reach your hands in front of you to rock forward. Your legs will elevate as you go.

pull the tailbone
toward the heels

lift the abs

18 Lift up your head and push back up to catch yourself on your hands. Your legs will descend. Rock forward and back for 5 more repetitions. Hold the last position to stabilize your body, then relax.

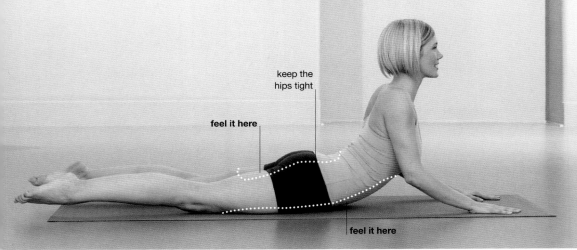

keep the
hips tight

feel it here

feel it here

19 Kneel on the floor and bend forward, stretching your arms along the floor above your head (see inset). Push back, allow your knees to open a little, then bring your hips back toward your heels. Place your palms one on top of the other underneath your forehead.

bring the hips
toward the heels

20 Inhale, push down on your hands, curl your head down, and round your back under, breathing in for 3 counts. Allow your hips to lift away from your feet a little. Bow your head and look toward your navel. Then exhale and lower your head and hips back toward the floor. Take 3 more in-and out-breaths as you perform this lifting and lowering motion.

let the hips lift

>> plank balance

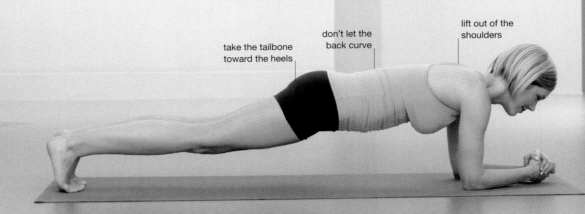

21 Go onto your forearms and knees, holding your hands together (see inset). Feel imaginary hands sandwiching your lower back (see p. 167). Exhale and reach your right foot behind you until your knee is straight, then reach your left foot behind you. Tuck your toes under to form 2 little stands. This is a forearm plank.

lift out of the shoulders

don't let the back curve

take the tailbone toward the heels

22 Exhale and balance on your left leg, pointing your toes of your right foot to the wall behind you. Breathe, then bring your right toes back under to the forearm plank position. Repeat to the other side, balancing on your right leg, then repeat to both sides once more.

lift the abs

>> "C" exercise

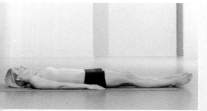

23 Lie on your back (see inset). Inhale, reach your arms up above your head on the floor, and clasp your hands. Stretch your ankles away from your head at the same time.

stretch the ankles away from the head

24 Slowly and smoothly slide your arms and legs to the right to make the letter "C" as seen from above. Repeat the body slide to the left. Feel as if your waist is lifting up and over an imaginary fence. Lengthen your body out, then repeat to the other side. Repeat another 4 times to right and left.

press the back onto the floor

15 minute

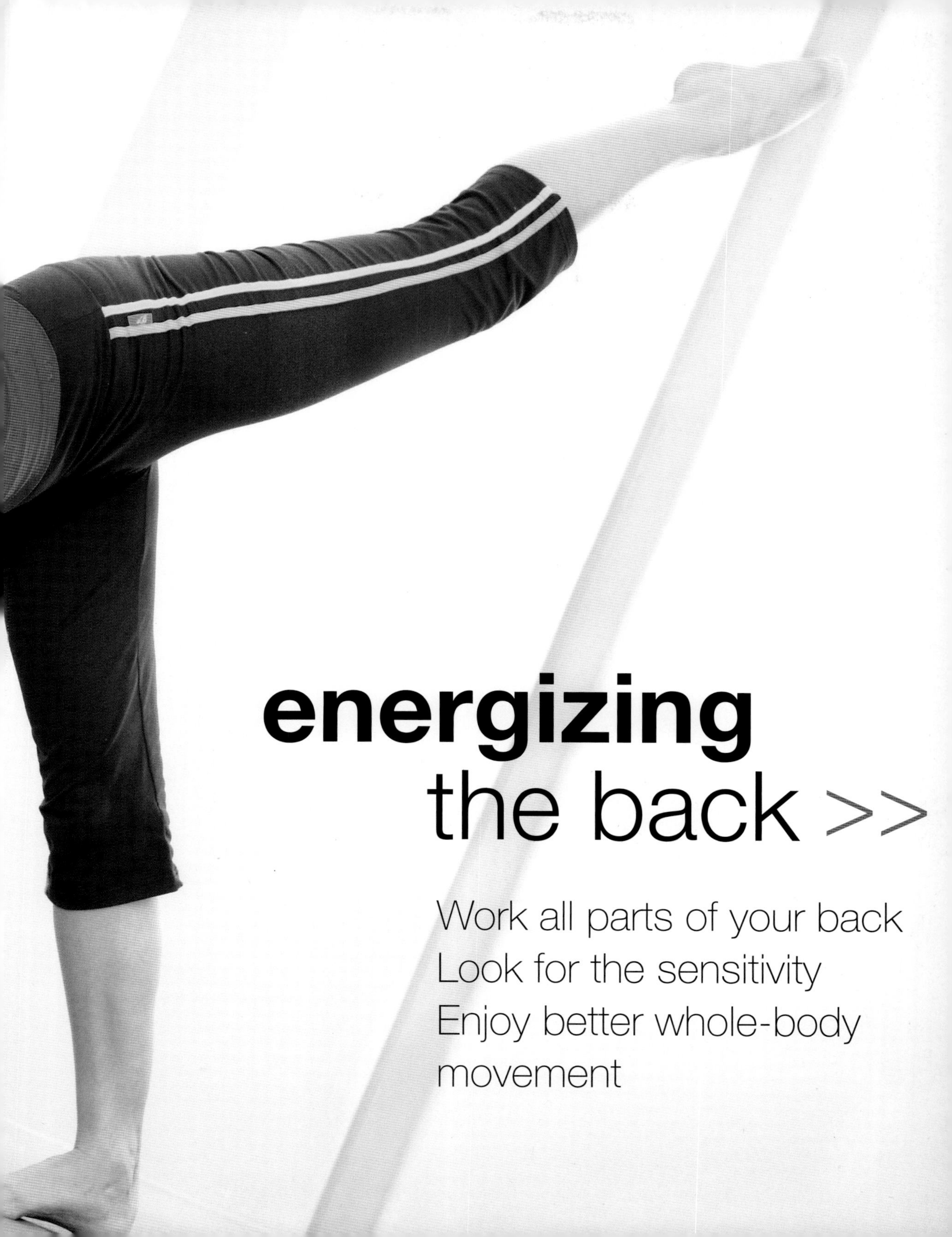

energizing
the back >>

Work all parts of your back
Look for the sensitivity
Enjoy better whole-body
movement

>> **arm circles**

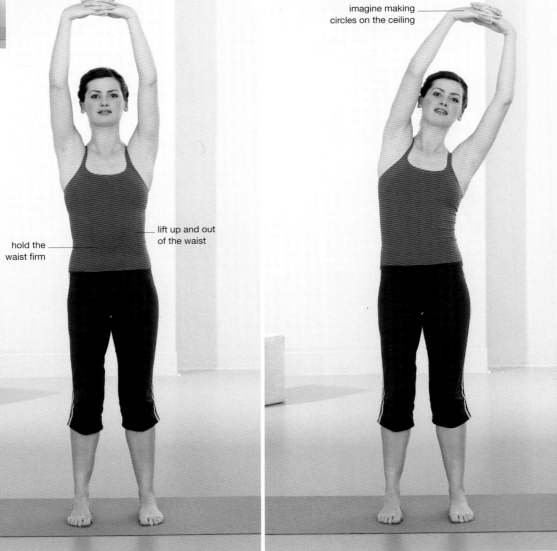

1 Stand with your legs shoulder-width apart (see inset). Reach both arms up overhead, and clasp your fingers. Lengthen your tailbone toward the ground. Circle your arms, imagining making 4 circles on the ceiling with your hands. Return to center.

2 Again, lift up and out of your waist and tighten your waist. Lengthen your tailbone. Reverse the movement with your hands, imagining making 4 more circles on the ceiling. Bring your arms down.

imagine making circles on the ceiling

lift up and out of the waist

hold the waist firm

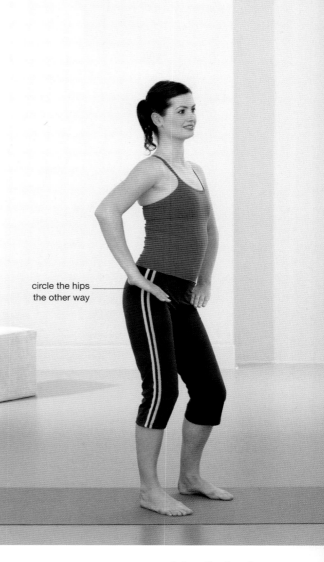

3 Stand with your legs about shoulder-width apart (see inset). Place your hands on your hips. Start moving your hips in a circling motion. Notice that your knees will also circle at the same time. Keep them a little bent. Be sure to tighten your waist. Circle your hips one way 5 times.

4 Still keeping your knees bent and your waist tight, circle your hips the other way 5 times. Repeat the hip circles again 5 times in each direction.

tighten the waist

keep the knees bent

circle the hips the other way

>> wrist and ankle circles

5 Stand with your legs about shoulder-width apart. Place your left hand on your left hip joint (see inset). Slowly shift onto your left leg, raise your right, and find your balance. Tighten in your waist to help with the balance or hold onto a chair. Press your left foot into the ground.

6 Circle your right ankle and right wrist at the same time. Circle 5 times. Reverse the direction for 5 circles. Repeat the whole exercise again, then shift onto your right leg and repeat, circling with the left foot and left hand. Take your left leg down to the floor.

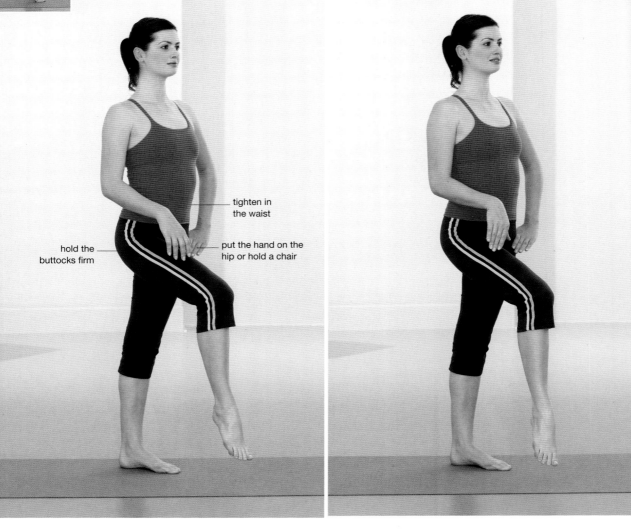

tighten in the waist

hold the buttocks firm

put the hand on the hip or hold a chair

>> **back stretch**

7 Stand tall with your feet just less than hip-width apart (see inset). Take your head over your pelvis (see p. 167). Pull your navel to your spine (see p. 167). Make fists with your hands and place your knuckles on your lower back. Exhale a little, then inhale as you lift your chest diagonally toward the ceiling.

8 Breathe, then return your chest and focus to look forward again by lifting through your ears. Repeat the exercise 3 more times, inhaling as you focus up toward the ceiling, and exhaling as you lengthen your spine and lift through your ears to return to look forward. As you lift your chest, feel as if a hook is pulling your breastbone up to the ceiling.

lift the chest to the ceiling

feel it here

lift through the ears to return

lift the abs toward the head

>> **side stretch 3**

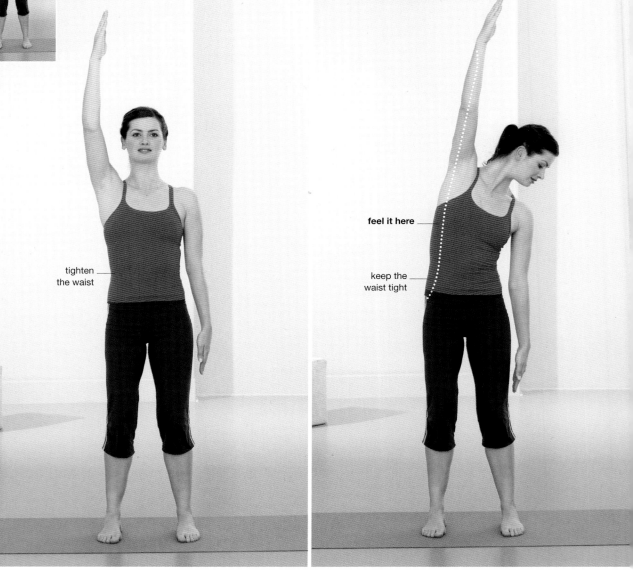

9 Stand with your feet hip-width apart (see inset). Pull your navel into your spine, drop your tailbone, and bend your knees slightly. Raise your right arm and pull your right middle finger to the ceiling.

10 Look down to the left and lean and pull your left middle finger toward the floor as you reach up with the right middle finger. Elongate the whole right side of your body. Lift your pelvis (see p. 167). Take 2 breaths and then return to center. Repeat on the other side. Return to center again.

tighten
the waist

feel it here

keep the
waist tight

11 Lie on your back with your knees bent and the soles of your feet on the floor. Your feet should be about shoulder-width apart (see inset). Place your hands on your pubic area and abdomen to feel the movement. Compress your back sequentially into the floor: first your pubic area, then your lower back, then your mid-back. Pull your navel to your spine as you go.

hollow the pubic area

12 Imagine you are pressing pearls into sand with your back (see p. 166) as you perform the exercise. End with a chin tuck. Hold for 4 counts, then repeat. Stretch your legs out onto the floor, and take your arms behind your head. Repeat the compressions 4 times. Relax.

tuck the chin

>> puppy dog abs

13 Lie on your back with your knees bent and arms by your sides (see inset). Hold your abs firm and lift your legs up so your shins are parallel to the floor. Bend your elbows, take your upper arms off the floor, and face your palms upward. This puppy dog position (see p. 167) makes your core muscles work.

take the upper arms off the floor

work the core muscles

14 Exhale, tilt your chin, lift your head, look to your groin, and lengthen your arms out past your hips. At the same time, reach your feet upward into a "V" shape, just past shoulder-width apart. Inhale and exhale, then lower back down to the puppy dog position. Repeat the exercise 3 more times.

look to the groin

>> **first position abs**

15 Lie on your back in first position parallel, with your second toe in line with your kneecaps and with the midpoint on your groin line (see p. 164). Flex your feet. Brace with your hands at your hip joint (see inset). Lift your head to check that you are in line. Keep your head up to start the exercise.

press the rib cage to the floor

brace the hands at the hips

press the thighs into the floor

point the knees upward

keep the lower back slightly off the floor

16 Exhale as you lower your head while dragging your legs to meet at the midline of your body. Firmly press your hips, knees, and ankles together, counting to 8. Repeat the lifting of your head with the opening of your legs, and the lowering of your head with pressing your legs together 3 more times. Finally, lift your head and open your legs. Relax down.

lower the head

press the legs together

drag the legs to the midline

>> **hip lift**

17 Lie on your right side with your right arm stretched out along the floor (see inset). Use your left hand for balance and lean up on your right forearm. Keep your legs together. Flex your feet hard and pull your toes up into your shins. Pull your navel to your spine. If balance is difficult, open your legs into a "V" shape.

press the hips forward

lean on the forearm

18 Inhale, then exhale and press downward on your legs as you look down and lift your pelvis off the floor. Hold for a moment, then lower, but not completely. Repeat 3 more times, then repeat lying on your left side.

feel it here

>> **swimming**

19 Lie on your front. Reach your hands above your head about shoulder-width apart on the floor, with your palms facing down and your arms slightly bent. Rest your forehead gently on the floor (see inset). Take your legs about 3 inches (7.5 cm) apart. Exhale, and levitate your head, hands, and feet about 2 inches (5 cm) off the floor.

pull the tailbone toward the heels

lift the abs

look downward

20 Keeping your torso as still as possible, start a small flutter-kick type of swimming motion with your feet. At the same time, "splash" alternately with your hands. Concentrate on not waddling from side to side. If your back tightens up, go down, breathe, rest, and then begin again. Work up to counting for 30 counts. Think: "1-Alligator, 2-Alligator," to set the rhythm. Relax down.

splash the hands

flutter kick the feet

1
 >> **inverted stretch**

keep the right hip low

21 Go onto all fours, then tuck your toes under and lift your knees off the floor to come up into an upside-down triangle. Touching your toes of your right foot to the floor (see inset), exhale, transfer almost all your weight into your right hand, and raise your right leg up behind you.

keep the leg parallel to the floor

22 Slowly open your right leg to your right side while keeping weight in your right hand. Press into your right hand as you return your foot behind you. Give your foot a little lift, lengthen, then lower. Repeat with your left leg.

>> hanging stretch

23 Stand with your legs about 3 inches (7.5 cm) apart. Place your left foot ahead of your right with about a foot's-width between your legs. Your toes point forward (see inset). Cross your arms, hold your elbows, and pull your navel firmly into your spine. Reach your elbows downward.

24 Continue to reach your elbows down toward the floor. Stay in this rounded position, firmly holding your abs as you take 3 breaths. Carefully roll up, feeling as if your abs are walking up the front of your body. Repeat on the other side. Come back up and relax.

look down the length of the body

lift the pelvic muscles

engage the hollow above the pubis

energizing the back at a glance

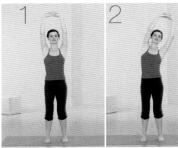
▲ Arm Circles, page 200

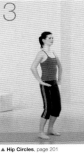
▲ Arm Circles, page 200

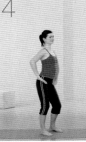
▲ Hip Circles, page 201

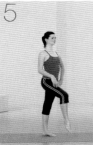
▲ Hip Circles, page 201

5 ▲ Wrist and Ankle Circles, page 202

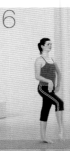
▲ Wrist and Ankle Circles, page 202

13 ▲ Puppy Dog Abs, page 206

14 ▲ Puppy Dog Abs, page 206

15 ▲ First Position Abs, page 207

16 ▲ First Position Abs, page 207

17 ▲ Hip Lift, page 208

18 ▲ Hip Lift, page 208

soothing the back at a glance

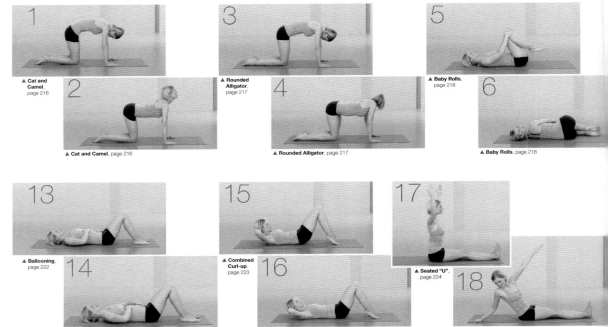

1 ▲ Cat and Camel, page 216

2 ▲ Cat and Camel, page 216

3 ▲ Rounded Alligator, page 217

4 ▲ Rounded Alligator, page 217

5 ▲ Baby Rolls, page 218

6 ▲ Baby Rolls, page 218

13 ▲ Ballooning, page 222

14 ▲ Ballooning, page 222

15 ▲ Combined Curl-up, page 223

16 ▲ Combined Curl-up, page 223

17 ▲ Seated "U", page 224

18 ▲ Seated "U", page 224

7

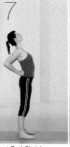

▲ **Back Stretch**, page 203

8

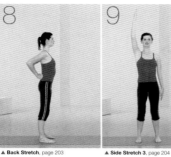

▲ **Back Stretch**, page 203

9

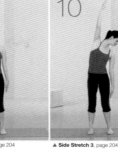

▲ **Side Stretch 3**, page 204

10

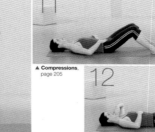

▲ **Side Stretch 3**, page 204

11

▲ **Compressions**, page 205

12

▲ **Compressions**, page 205

19

▲ **Swimming**, page 209

20

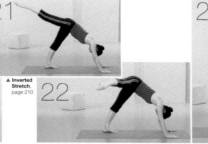

▲ **Swimming**, page 209

21

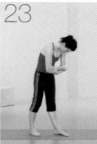

▲ **Inverted Stretch**, page 210

22

▲ **Inverted Stretch**, page 210

23

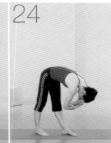

▲ **Hanging Stretch**, page 211

24

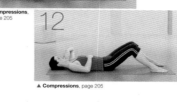

▲ **Hanging Stretch**, page 211

7

▲ **Sacral Circles**, page 219

8

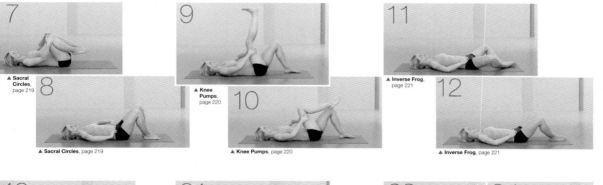

▲ **Sacral Circles**, page 219

9

▲ **Knee Pumps**, page 220

10

▲ **Knee Pumps**, page 220

11

▲ **Inverse Frog**, page 221

12

▲ **Inverse Frog**, page 221

19

▲ **Heel Taps**, page 225

20

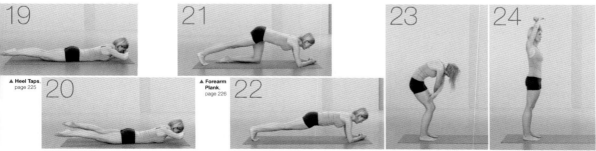

▲ **Heel Taps**, page 225

21

▲ **Forearm Plank**, page 226

22

▲ **Forearm Plank**, page 226

23

▲ **Hangover Roll-up**, page 227

24

▲ **Hangover Roll-up**, page 227

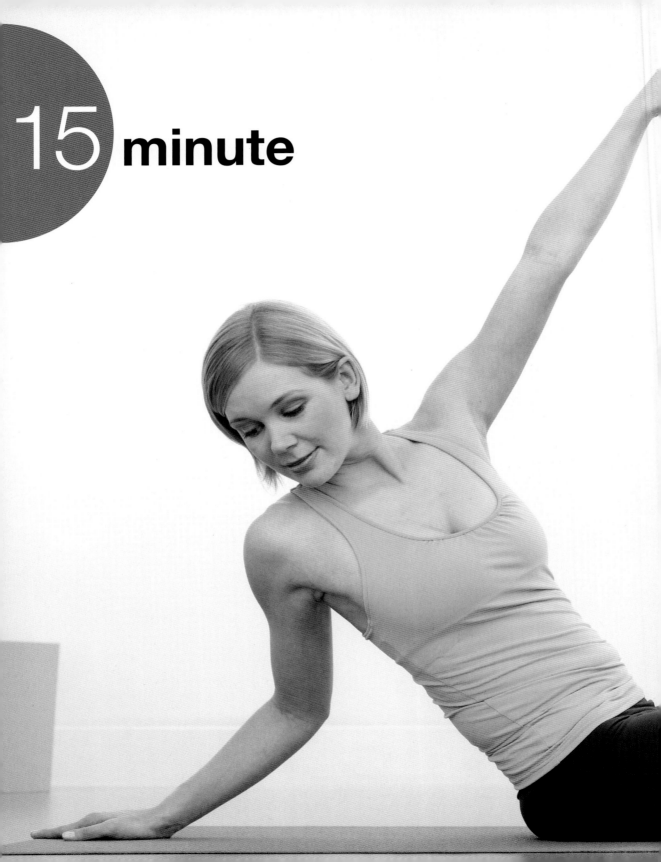

15 minute

Think supple and lithe,
smooth and flowing
Fluidity means grace
and ease

soothing
the back >>

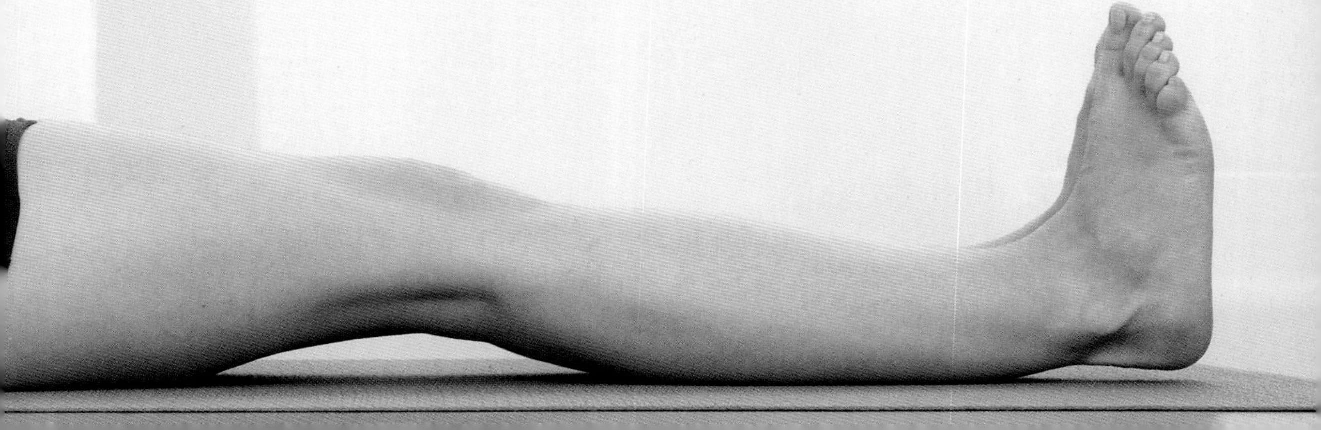

>> **cat and camel**

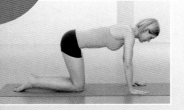

1 Start on all fours with your back flat in the tabletop position (see p. 166). Lengthen out from your tailbone as though you have a long tail (see inset). Then reach out through your head and tilt your chin and tailbone down at the same time. Round your back to look at your navel, like a scared cat.

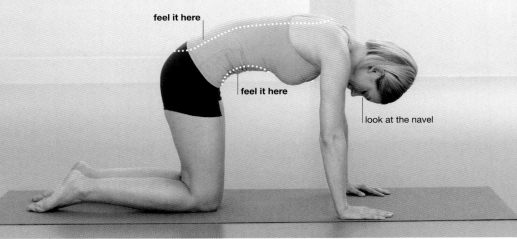

feel it here

feel it here

look at the navel

2 Exhale and lengthen back to the tabletop, then look forward and arch your back like a camel by reaching up and out through your head. Feel as if your tailbone could reach the top of your head. Repeat the exercise 1 more time. Return to the tabletop position and relax.

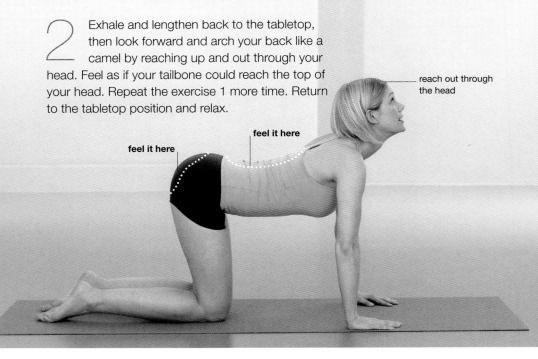

reach out through the head

feel it here

feel it here

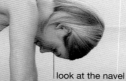

3 Remain on all fours and look toward your right hip. Swing your right hip toward your right shoulder. Now round your back and look at your navel as in the scared cat position (see opposite).

look at the navel

4 Repeat the exercise to look at your left hip, while swinging your left hip toward your left shoulder. Round your back again and look at your navel. Repeat 2 more times.

swing the left hip to the left shoulder

>> **baby rolls**

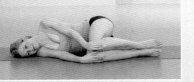

5 Start by lying on your right side with your legs bent up. Hold your hands on top of your knees (see inset). Put a towel around your neck if you need extra support. Roll onto your back, feeling as much of your back as possible resting against the floor.

don't tilt the chin

feel it here | feel the back against the floor

6 Then roll over onto your left side, letting your focus and head linger to the right. Think: "leg, leg," then your head rolls last. Repeat the exercise, starting on your left side, then rolling onto your back, and lingering the focus to the left. Continue gently rolling from side to side 3 more times.

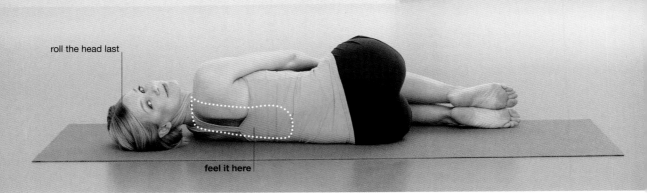

roll the head last

feel it here

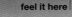

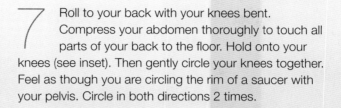

7 Roll to your back with your knees bent. Compress your abdomen thoroughly to touch all parts of your back to the floor. Hold onto your knees (see inset). Then gently circle your knees together. Feel as though you are circling the rim of a saucer with your pelvis. Circle in both directions 2 times.

compress the abdomen | circle the pelvis

8 Place the soles of your feet on the floor. Keep your knees bent. Place your hands on your hip bones for feedback. Circle your pelvis again as before. Move in one direction for 4 circles, then reverse. Circle your pelvis 2 more times in each direction.

place the hands on the hip bones

>> knee pumps

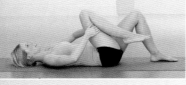

pull the toes
toward the shin

feel it here

9 Stay on your back. Bend both knees. Take your feet about 4 inches (10 cm) apart. Lift up your right leg and use both hands to hold loosely behind your lifted thigh (see inset). Then gently straighten your knee. It does not have to straighten completely. At the top of the stretch, pull your toes toward your shin.

10 Still holding onto your thigh, bend your knee, letting your foot come down so your shin makes a parallel line with the floor. Perform this pumping action 10 times. Repeat the exercise holding your left leg. Relax.

bring the shin
parallel with the floor

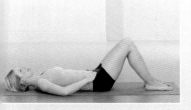

11 Stay on your back with bent knees. Compress your whole back against the floor and place your hands on your hips for feedback (see inset). Keep your back pressed firmly against the floor as you gently open both knees sideways toward the floor, like a frog. Let the soles of your feet come together.

place the hands
on the hip bones

soles of the feet
come together

feel the back against the floor

12 Exhale and deepen the abdominal compression as you bring the knees together again. Repeat the frog-like opening and closing 3 more times. Relax.

bring the
knees together

compress the
abdomen

press the lower back against the floor

>> **ballooning**

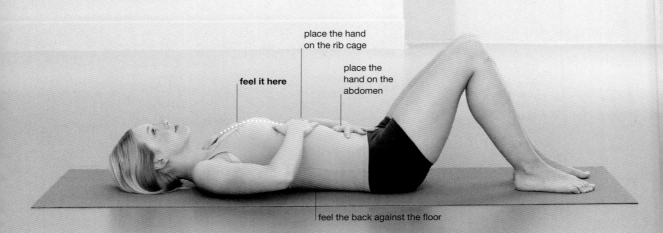

13 Stay on your back with knees bent. Let your whole back fall into the floor. Place your left hand on your abdomen, and your right hand on your rib cage with your thumb between your breasts (see inset). Breathe in through your nose. Expand your chest and tighten your abs.

place the hand on the rib cage

place the hand on the abdomen

feel it here

feel the back against the floor

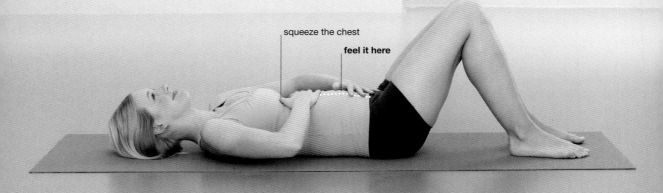

14 Now reverse the action. Breathe out through your mouth, squeeze your chest, and expand your abs. Inhale, expand your chest; exhale, and squeeze your chest, for 3 more repetitions. Think of mercury in a thermometer flowing up and down the front of your spine as you perform this exercise.

squeeze the chest

feel it here

>> **combined curl-up**

15 Stay on your back with knees bent and heels lifted, a little apart. Clasp your hands behind your head (see inset). Simultaneously tilt your chin, curl your upper body off the floor to look at your groin, and tuck and roll your tailbone off the floor. Imagine a dog's tail between your legs, lifting your tailbone and spine (see p. 167).

imagine keeping the ribs below the tailbone

16 Take a breath, then lower your head, shoulders, and tailbone back down to the ground at the same time. Keep your heels up off the floor. Imagine you are pressing pearls into sand with your spine (see p. 166). Repeat the Combined Curl-up 2 more times.

keep the elbows out

keep the heels up

>> seated "U"

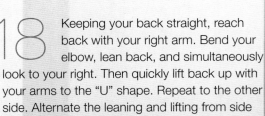

17 Sit up tall on your sitbones with both legs extended straight out in front of you (see inset). Feel an imaginary hand lifting the skin of your lower back up and toward your head. Then pull your toes up toward your shins, exhale, and levitate your hands to make a "U" shape.

drop the shoulders down

reach out with the top hand

18 Keeping your back straight, reach back with your right arm. Bend your elbow, lean back, and simultaneously look to your right. Then quickly lift back up with your arms to the "U" shape. Repeat to the other side. Alternate the leaning and lifting from side to side for 3 more sets.

>> **heel taps**

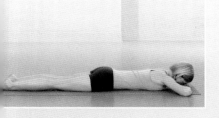

19 Lie on your front with outstretched legs. Place your hands underneath your forehead, and rest your head on top (see inset). Rotate your legs to a "V" shape, heels together and toes apart. Exhale as you levitate your head, hands, and feet about 2 inches (5 cm) off the floor. Feel the smile lines (see p. 166). Look downward.

take the tailbone
toward the heels

lift the abs

20 Tap your heels together a total of 32 times, in 4 sets of 8. Frequently improve the work of the exercise by holding your abs inward and tight, anchoring your hips with a strong tailbone tuck, and pulling the gaze toward the floor. End by holding and tightening your hips, then lower down and relax.

regularly check that
the abs are tight

>> **forearm plank**

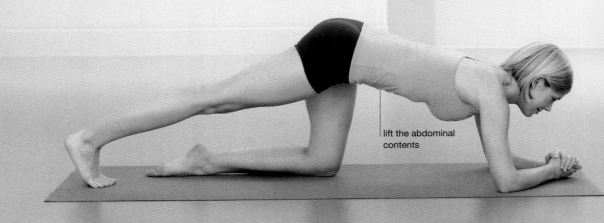

21 Go onto your forearms and knees. Clasp your hands in front of you (see inset). Feel imaginary hands sandwiching your waist (see p. 167). One lifts your abdominal contents and the other gently presses down on your lower back. Inhale and exhale to reach your right foot and then the left behind you to create a Forearm Plank.

lift the abdominal contents

22 Pull up your abs and press your pubic bone down toward the floor. Curl your tailbone under to firmly lock in your hips. Take 2 breaths. Bend your knees back to kneeling, then repeat the exercise. Relax.

pull up the abs

>> **hangover roll-up**

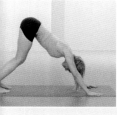

23 From all fours, exhale and lift your hips (see inset), holding your navel to your spine (see p. 167). Walk your hands toward your feet. Keep your knees a little bent. Take 2 breaths, then start rolling up. As you pass your thighs, cross your wrists and take off an imaginary shirt.

24 Continue rolling up, feeling as if the vertebrae are stacking up vertically through your lower back, waistline, rib cage, and shoulders, until your head reaches up on top of your pelvis (see p. 167). Circle your arms to lower. Relax.

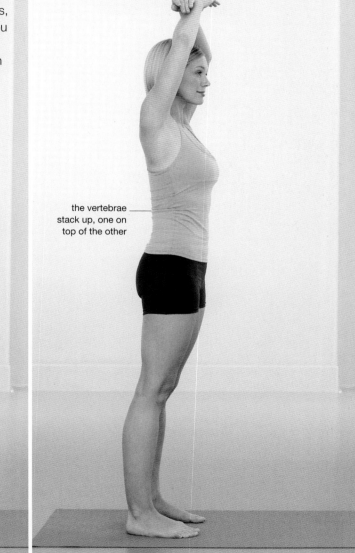

the vertebrae stack up, one on top of the other

feel how the head becomes heavy

feel how the tailbone becomes heavy

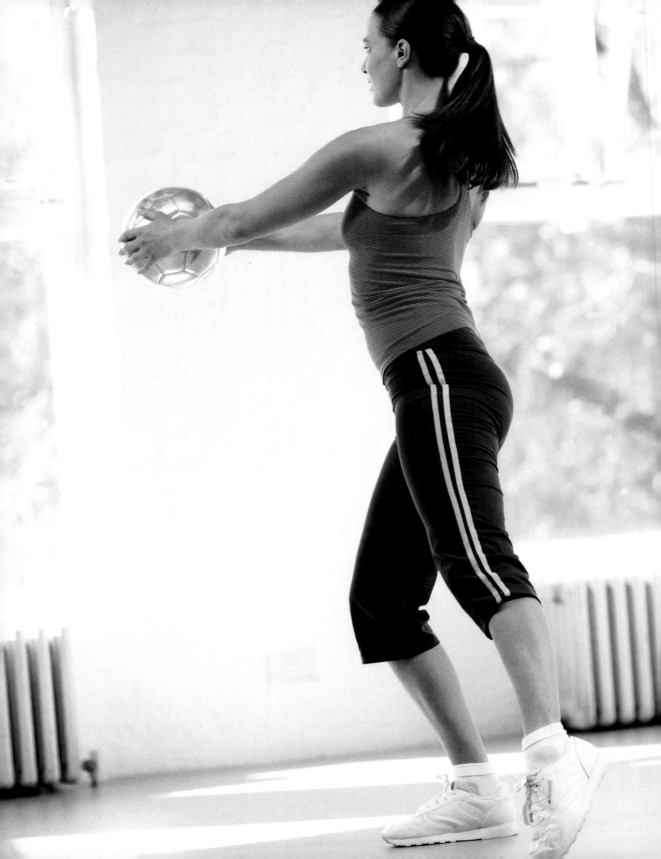

total body
workout

Joan Pagano

>> working the total body

No more excuses! It's time to get moving. Do you think you're too busy, can't afford it, or don't have enough room or equipment to work out at home? Maybe you feel it's too boring, not fun, and you can't stick with it? Or that you're too lazy, old, fat, or out of shape to even begin?

The list of excuses not to get fit is endless, but the solution is simple: *Total Body Workout* provides the tools you need for an exercise program with minimal investment of time and resources, and from which you will definitely benefit.

15-minute workouts

The *Total Body Workout* exercise routines are designed to give you maximum benefit in the most efficient format, combining cardio and strength training. All it takes to complete a full-body routine is 15 minutes. Therefore, if 15 minutes is all you have, pick just one of them. Or, if you have more time, combine the routines for a 30-, 45-, or 60-minute workout. Choose your workout according to your level of fitness, energy, and available time.

Each of the four 15-minute workouts has a unique theme to make it more enjoyable and offer variety to your routines. They all challenge your body in different ways: Step-Touch (see p. 238) eases you into the habit of exercising. Toning Ball (see p. 256) uses a ball in a variety of sporty moves. Hop, Jig, and Jump (see p. 272) evokes the childlike joy of jumping. Lunge Around the Clock (see p. 290) requires the most skill and tests your limits a little bit more.

The formula for each workout is consistent: a three-minute warm up, 10 minutes of strength (or resistance) training exercises alternating with cardio intervals, and a two-minute cool down. These workouts have been selected to maximize your results by impacting all aspects of fitness.

>> SMART tips for success

Goal setting is one of the best ways to stay motivated to exercise. The SMART system states that goals should be:

- **Specific** What exactly do you want to achieve? Reduce fat, improve muscle tone, increase bone density? With clear goals, you can choose appropriate exercises.

- **Measurable** Unless your goal is measurable, you won't know if you've accomplished it. Specific goals are measurable: muscle tone can be measured by endurance exercises.

- **Action-oriented** An action plan breaking your long-term goal into weekly targets will give you the satisfaction of meeting short-term goals, and the opportunity to reassess whether your goals are reasonable.

- **Realistic** People often become disillusioned and stop exercising when they don't get their imagined results. Are your goals in sync with your body type? Do they match your personal preferences?

- **Timed** Setting a target date gives you the motivation to stick with an exercise program, but you must allow a realistic amount of time to achieve your goal.

Composition of a workout

The warm ups are a series of movements that gradually build in intensity, giving you the flavor of the workout and preparing your body for the exercises to come. The strength-training programs comply with fitness industry guidelines that target the major muscles of the hips, thighs, legs, back, chest, shoulders, arms, and abdomen. The one-minute cardio intervals carry out the theme of the workout, at a higher level of intensity to pump up your heart in between the resistance exercises.

The body of the workout is composed of standing exercises for the purpose of burning more calories and preserving bone density. Many of them are combination moves involving multiple muscle groups, such as Lunge and Row (see p. 265), and Squat with Knee Lift (see p. 264). Again, the purpose is to produce the best results for your efforts: to target the most muscle groups, burn the most calories, and improve coordination at the same time; training your muscles to work in patterns.

No workout is complete without a full-body stretch, and this is provided in the cool down. As opposed to more traditional stretches that isolate individual muscles, these positions target multiple muscle groups, often stretching the upper and lower body together. They provide a fluid sequence as you progress through the movements.

Integrating all of these aspects of training prepares your whole body to meet the demands of your day-to-day activities more effectively (i.e. functional training). You'll really appreciate it the next time you are walking home on a wet, windy day, an open umbrella in one hand, a tote bag over the opposite shoulder, with several shopping bags in the other hand, when you want to buy a newspaper without falling over. This is the payoff of functional training.

To obtain maximum benefit and prevent injury, careful attention to form and posture is essential when exercising.

tools of the trade: clipboard and stopwatch

>> **your training** program

Now that you've assessed your current condition, you are ready to start making improvements to your personal level of fitness, as well as your health, appearance, energy levels, and overall mood. Each 15-minute workout combines cardio with resistance training and stretching.

Cardiovascular stamina, muscular strength and endurance, flexibility, and body composition are the aspects of physical fitness that are most closely related to health. Each of these characteristics is directly related to good health and to your risk of developing certain types of disease—notably those that are associated with inactivity.

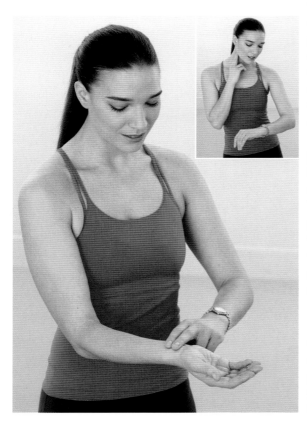

Benefits of cardiovascular fitness

A fit cardiovascular system is associated with a stronger heart muscle, slower heart rate, decreased chance of heart attack, and a greater chance of surviving if you do suffer a heart attack. Regular aerobic exercise can reduce your blood pressure and blood fats, including low-density lipids (LDL), which can help you resist build up of plaque in the arteries (atherosclerosis). It can also increase the protective high-density lipids (HDL) and improve circulation and the capacity of the blood to carry oxygen throughout your body. Improving cardiovascular fitness also decreases your risk of some cancers and of obesity, diabetes, osteoporosis, depression, and anxiety.

With training, your heart gets stronger and can pump more blood with each beat, resulting in a lower heart rate during exercise and at rest. The average resting rate is 60 to 80 beats per minute. Take your resting heart rate when you start your program and then eight weeks later and compare the numbers. Find your pulse (see left), count the first beat as "zero" and time yourself for 30 seconds. Multiply the score by two to arrive at the number of beats per minute.

Taking your pulse To take your pulse at the wrist (the "radial pulse") place your index and middle fingers on the palm side of the opposite wrist. Alternatively, you can take your pulse at the neck (the "carotid pulse"), just below the jaw bone to the side of the larynx.

Muscle strength and endurance

Muscular strength (the ability to exert force) and endurance (the ability of the muscles to exert themselves repeatedly) allow you to work more efficiently and to resist fatigue, muscle soreness, and back problems. Strengthening the muscles and joints allows you to increase the intensity and duration of your cardiovascular training. As you work the muscles, you simultaneously stimulate the bones to build and maintain density, decreasing the risk of developing osteoporosis.

Stretching and flexibility

Your ability to stretch out the muscles and maintain range of motion in the joints is another aspect of muscular fitness. Stretching helps improve posture by correcting the tendency of certain muscles to shorten and tighten; it counteracts the physical stressors of our day-to-day activities and discharges tension from the muscles.

Frequency and duration

For resistance training you need to do a minimum of two 15-minute sessions per week, and no muscle should be worked more than three times in one week. Allow a day of rest in between working each muscle group, since the repair and recovery of the muscle fibers is as important as the stress to the development of the muscle. The length of your session will vary from 15 to 60 minutes, depending on your initial fitness and available time.

Maintenance program

Periodically, you should vary the workouts you choose or the order you perform them in so that you keep your muscles "alert." You may also want to increase your weights (see pp. 236–237 for equipment), but be aware that this may trigger problems in the neck, shoulder, elbow, low back, or knee. You may be able to handle heavier weights in some muscle groups, but not in others, so experiment carefully. Posture and alignment, and core conditioning are also important aspects of your training.

>> myths about weight training

● **Myth 1**
Lifting weights will make you bulk up.

Truth Only if you have high levels of testosterone and use very heavy weights. Most women lack the necessary hormones and strength to build significant muscle mass.

● **Myth 2**
You shouldn't lift weights if you are an older adult, overweight, or out of shape.

Truth Not so! Weight training can help you rejuvenate, lose weight, and shape up.

● **Myth 3**
A thin person does not need to build lean body mass by lifting weights.

Truth Appearances are deceiving when it comes to body composition, and being thin is no guarantee that you are lean. Without weight training, you steadily lose muscle and gain fat as you age.

● **Myth 4**
Certain weight-training exercises can help you spot reduce.

Truth You can spot strengthen and shape a body area, but fat belongs to the whole body and needs to be reduced all over, through expending more calories (aerobic exercise and weight training) than you consume.

● **Myth 5**
Aerobic activities, not weight training, are the most efficient type of exercise to lose weight.

Truth Losing weight requires a balanced exercise program of aerobic exercise to burn calories and weight training to speed up the metabolism.

>> **anatomy** of an exercise

If you know which muscle is working in a particular exercise, you can enhance your effort by mentally focusing on it. This will help you key into the muscular movement and improve your body awareness.

CHEST
Pectorals
Half Push-up and Side
Plank, p. 303

ARMS
Biceps
Lunge and Curl, p. 247
Squat with Weight Shift, p. 266
Plié and Curl, p. 282
Lift and Squat, p. 301

ABDOMEN
Obliques
Bicycle Crunch,p. 251
Plank, p. 250, p. 271
Lunge and Twist, pp. 279-280
Half Push-up and Side Plank, p. 303

Rectus abdominis
Bicycle Crunch, p. 251
Plank, p. 250, p. 271
Half Push-up and Side Plank, p. 303

Transversus abdominis
Bicycle Crunch, p. 251

OUTER THIGH
Hip abductor
Lateral Lift, p. 283

FRONT OF THIGH
Quadriceps
Plié with Lateral Raise, p. 243
Lunge and Curl, p. 247
Squat, p. 248
Plié with Front Raise, p. 261
Squat with Knee Lift, p. 264
Lunge and Row, p. 265
Squat with Weight Shift, p. 266
Lunge and Twist, pp. 279-280
Side-Squat Jump, p. 281
Balance and Press, p. 282
Plié and Curl, p. 282
Wood-Chop Squat, p. 295
Plié and Row, p. 299
Balance Squat, p. 299
Lift and Squat, p. 301

Muscle groups and corresponding exercises
The anatomical illustrations will help you target specific areas that you want to work on.

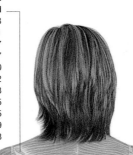

SHOULDER
Deltoid
Plié with Lateral Raise, p. 243
Plié with Front Raise, p. 261
Reverse Fly, p. 267
Hip Hinge and Reverse Fly, p. 277
Lunge and Twist, pp. 279-280
Balance and Press, p. 282
Lateral Lift, p. 283
Arm and Leg Lift, p. 285
Wood-Chop Squat, p. 295
Plié and Row, p. 299
Half Push-up and Side Plank, p. 303

ARMS
Triceps
Triceps Kick Back, p. 248
Triceps Double
Kick Back, p. 267
Lift and Squat, p. 301
Half Push-up
and Side Plank, p. 303

BUTTOCKS
Gluteals/Glutes
Plié with Lateral Raise, p. 243
Lunge and Curl, p. 247
Squat, p. 248
Plié with Front Raise, p. 261
Squat with Knee Lift, p. 264
Lunge and Row, p. 265
Squat with Weight Shift, p. 266
Hip Hinge and
Reverse Fly, p. 277
Lunge and Twist, pp. 279-280
Side Squat Jump, p. 281
Plié and Curl, p. 282
Arm and Leg Lift, p. 285
Wood-Chop Squat, p. 295
Plié and Row, p. 299
Balance Squat, p. 299
Lift and Squat, p. 301

BACK OF THIGH
Hamstrings
Plié with Lateral Raise, p. 243
Lunge and Curl, p. 247
Squat, p. 248
Plié with Front Raise, p. 261
Squat with Knee Lift, p. 264
Lunge and Row, p. 265
Squat with Weight Shift, p. 266
Hip Hinge and
Reverse Fly, p. 277
Lunge and Twist, pp. 279-280
Side Squat Jump, p. 281
Plié and Curl, p. 282
Wood-Chop Squat, p. 295
Plié and Row, p. 299
Balance Squat, p. 299
Lift and Squat, p. 301

>>**the main** muscle groups

- **Hips and thighs** (gluteals, quadriceps, hamstrings, and hip adductors and abductors)
- **Back** (latissimus dorsi, rhomboids, trapezius, and erector spinae)
- **Chest** (pectorals)
- **Shoulders** (deltoids)
- **Arms** (biceps and triceps)
- **Abdomen** (rectus abdominis, transversus abdominis, and obliques)

BACK
Rhomboids & Trapezius
Bent-over Row, p. 300

Latissimus dorsi
One-arm Row, p. 247
Lunge and Row, p. 265
Lunge and Twist, pp. 279-280
Bent-over Row, p.300

Erector spinae
Arm and Leg Lift, p. 285

INNER THIGH
Hip adductor
Plié with Lateral Raise, p. 243
Plié with Front Raise, p. 261
Plié and Curl, p. 282
Plié and Row, p. 299

LOWER LEG, CALF
Squat with Weight Shift, p. 266
Side-Squat Jump, p. 281
Lift and Squat, p. 301

>> **equipment** and clothing

I recommend a ball and two pairs of free weights (also called hand weights, or dumbbells), either 3 lb (1 kg) and 5 lb (2 kg), or 5 lb (2 kg) and 8 lb (4 kg), depending on your starting level. An exercise mat is also useful to provide cushioning as well as traction for some of the exercises.

My preferences and recommendations in your choices of equipment are based on quality, economy, and safety of use.

What to wear

Wear comfortable clothing that you can move in; some people prefer formfitting clothing because it makes it easier to monitor body alignment, while others prefer less-revealing loose clothing. Shoes, for example cross-trainers, should be supportive and allow movement in all directions. Running shoes are not a good choice as they are designed primarily for moving forward and backward only.

Free weights

These make resistance training interesting by challenging your balance, coordination, and core stabilization. Since you lift them with individual limbs, it is easy to spot imbalances in the body and to use them to improve symmetry. You can effectively isolate one muscle at a time, or combine movements to challenge whole muscle groups. Free weights are usually solid metal covered in gray

Free weights and balls come in a variety of sizes and finishes. Both weights and balls should be comfortable to hold and easy to use.

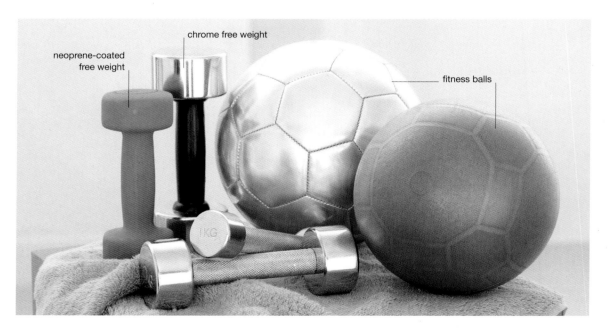

neoprene-coated free weight

chrome free weight

fitness balls

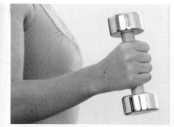

Holding the weight, make sure to keep your wrist flat to prevent any strain or injury to the joint.

Picking up weights
1 Kneel down. Keep your back straight and tighten your abdominals as you prepare to lift the weights.

2 Use the large muscles in your legs to do the lifting, squeezing your glutes as you stand up. Keep working your abdominals to protect your lower back.

enamel, chrome, vinyl, neoprene (which contains latex), or rubber. Enamel and chrome coatings chip and flake over time, presenting a small risk. Some people prefer neoprene-coated weights as they are nicer to hold, and do not become slippery with sweat. Free weights are widely available in various weight increments.

Balls

A simple, unweighted beach ball will do just fine, but a weighted "medicine" ball provides resistance for muscle toning. My personal favorites are filled with gel and feel good to the touch. I recommend a weight of 3 lb (1 kg) or 4 lb (1.5 kg) because anything heavier may cause strain in the neck and

shoulders from repetitive motions. A convenient size to fit in your hands is 7–10 in (18–25 cm) in diameter, although smaller balls will work too. Anything larger than this might be too unwieldy.

Exercise mats

Exercise mats are readily available in a variety of different densities of foam that either fold or roll up. Of the foldable mats, I prefer the dense foam, which is stiff to touch but surprisingly resilient to use. Of the roll-up mats, I prefer a soft durable foam because it offers comfortable cushioning with a sticky surface to prevent sliding. A yoga "sticky mat" is great for this too, but doesn't offer the same degree of cushioning.

15 minute

step-touch
workout >>

Gently ease yourself into the habit of exercising with this lighter workout

>> march/heel dig

1 To begin your warm up, stand with your feet parallel, hip width apart, knees soft, arms by your sides. Begin marching, bending one knee to bring the foot just off the floor and swinging the opposite arm forward and other arm back. Step down on the ball of your foot, rolling through to the heel. Continue marching, using opposite arm/leg action. Repeat for a total of 8 reps (1 rep = both sides).

2 Continuing to march, change the foot pattern to a heel dig to the front. Extend your leg to the front, knee straight, heel to the floor, toe to the ceiling. Continue to pump the arms in opposition as you march, with elbows bent close to your sides, raising the front fist to shoulder height. Remember to keep your abs pulled tight. Repeat for a total of 8 reps (1 rep = both sides).

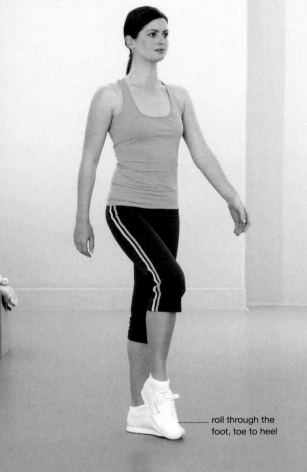

roll through the foot, toe to heel

hold the hands in loose fists

place the heel to the floor, point toe to ceiling

3 Change the foot pattern to a toe reach to the front and continue marching, alternating feet and arms. As you extend your leg, point the foot, lengthening from toe to hip. Keep your arms straight as you swing them, raising the front hand to shoulder height. As you work, focus on your alignment. Stack your shoulders over your hips, over your ankles. Look straight ahead. Repeat the Toe Reach for a total of 8 reps (1 rep = both sides).

4 Step up the intensity by bending the front knee to hip height. If you are able to lift the knee higher than your hip, be sure to use your core muscles to maintain proper alignment. Continue to pump the arms in opposition, raising the front elbow to shoulder level. Repeat the Knee Raise for a total of 8 reps (1 rep = both sides).

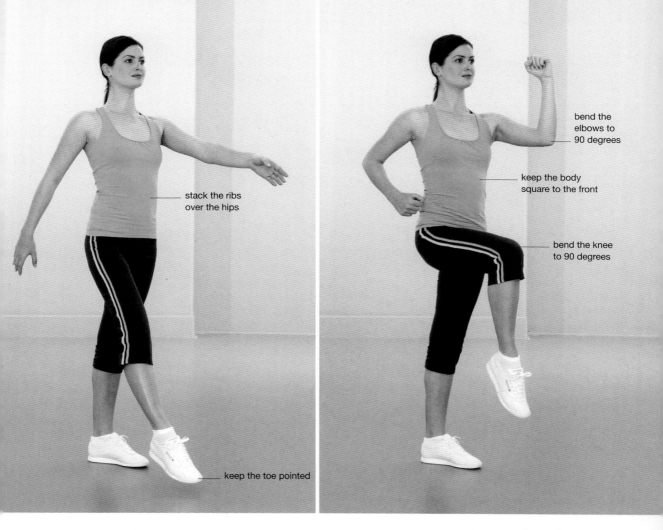

stack the ribs over the hips

keep the toe pointed

bend the elbows to 90 degrees

keep the body square to the front

bend the knee to 90 degrees

>> reverse lunge/lateral lift

5 Maintaining the same rhythm, bend one leg and extend the the other leg behind, heel raised. Raise both arms to the front at shoulder height. Push off with the ball of your back foot to return to center, arms returning to your sides, then switch sides and repeat. Repeat the Reverse Lunge for a total of 8 reps (1 rep = both sides).

6 Maintaining the same rhythm, bend both knees, arms by your sides. Then straighten both legs, lift one leg to the side and raise both arms to shoulder level. Return the raised leg to center, knees bent. Repeat, alternating sides, for 8 reps (1 rep = both sides). Now **reverse**, starting with step 5, and working back through steps 4, 3, and 2, and finishing with step 1, marching in place to finish your warm up.

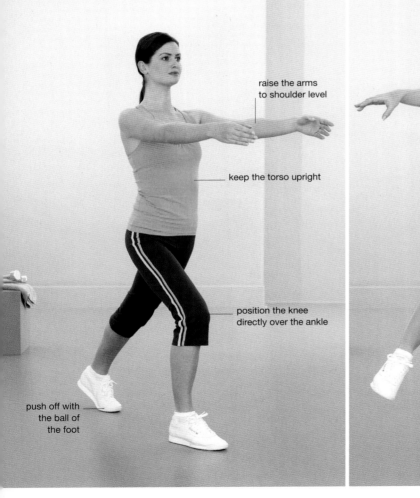

raise the arms
to shoulder level

keep the torso upright

position the knee
directly over the ankle

push off with
the ball of
the foot

knees bend
and straighten

>> plié with lateral raise

7a Pick up two small free weights and stand with your feet in a wide stance. Shift your weight to your heels and turn your legs out from the hips as a unit until your feet are at 45 degree angles. Hold the free weights with palms facing in, arms straight by your sides. Remember to pull your abdominals tight and draw your shoulder blades down and together.

7b Inhale as you bend your knees in line with your feet, lifting your arms out to the sides to shoulder height, thumbs up to the ceiling. Angle your arms slightly forward of your body, directly above your thighs. Keep your elbows slightly rounded and your wrists straight. Exhale and press through your heels as you straighten your legs and lower your arms to return to the start position. As you move, imagine you are sliding up and down a wall. Repeat for a total of 12 reps.

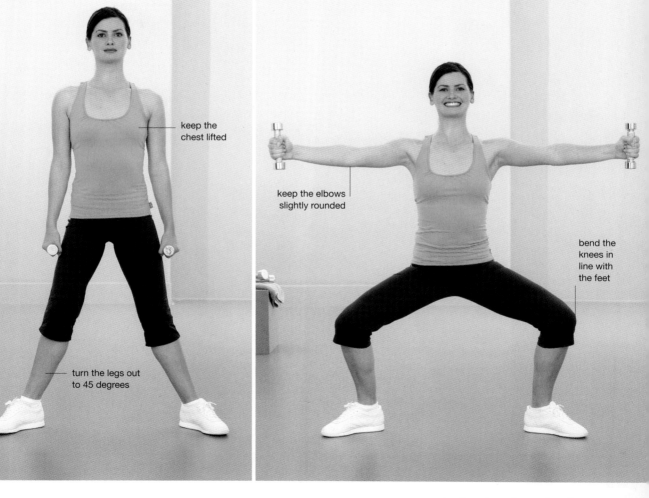

keep the chest lifted

turn the legs out to 45 degrees

keep the elbows slightly rounded

bend the knees in line with the feet

>> **step and punch**

8a Put down the weights for the first cardio interval. Stand with your feet parallel, shoulder width apart, knees bent in a demi plié. Bend your arms and hold them at shoulder height, hands in loose fists. Check your alignment: keep your shoulder blades down, abs tight, chest lifted, and torso square to the front.

8b Breathe in, then exhale as you straighten your knees and extend one arm diagonally across your body (like a punch), at the same time lifting the heel of the same leg. Keep your other arm bent at shoulder height. Inhale as you return to the start position and repeat, alternating sides, for 12 reps (1 rep = both sides).

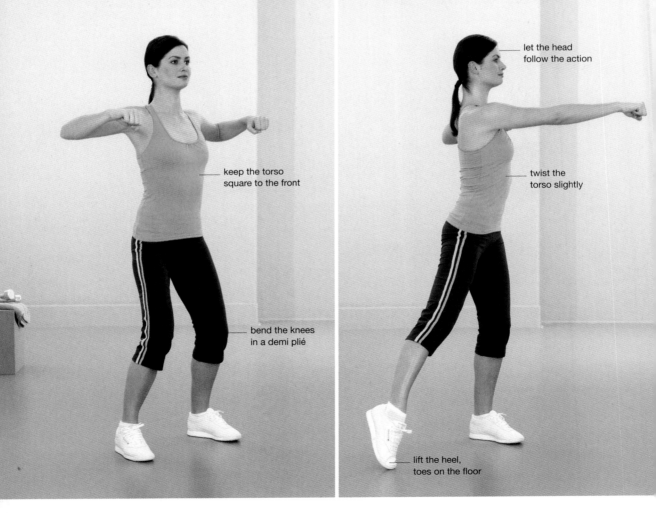

keep the torso
square to the front

bend the knees
in a demi plié

let the head
follow the action

twist the
torso slightly

lift the heel,
toes on the floor

>> **curl and squeeze**

9a Stand with your feet parallel, shoulder width apart, knees soft. Raise your arms to the front at shoulder level, shoulder width apart, hands in loose fists, palms down. Keep your knees soft. Use your core muscles to maintain neutral spine alignment, and lower your shoulder blades as you prepare to work the muscles of the mid-back.

9b Breathing naturally throughout, shift your weight onto one leg and simultaneously bend the other leg back, heel toward your buttocks, in a hamstring curl. Keep your arms parallel to the floor, elbows bent at 90 degrees, as you squeeze your shoulder blades together. Inhale as you return to the starting position. Repeat, alternating legs, for a total of 8 reps (1 rep = both sides).

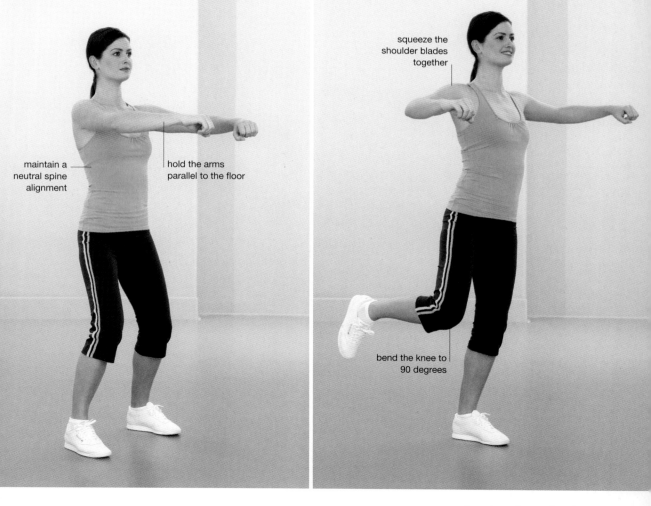

maintain a neutral spine alignment

hold the arms parallel to the floor

squeeze the shoulder blades together

bend the knee to 90 degrees

>> **twisting knee lift**

10a Stand with your feet parallel, hip-width apart, knees soft. Raise your arms out to the sides at shoulder height and bend your elbows to 90 degrees; with palms facing forward, make your hands into loose fists. Remember to keep your shoulder blades down and abs pulled tight as you get ready to twist.

10b Keeping your back straight, bend your knee to hip height. Exhale and rotate your torso through the center to bring your elbow toward your raised knee. Inhale as you return to the center and repeat, alternating sides, for 8 reps (1 rep = both sides).

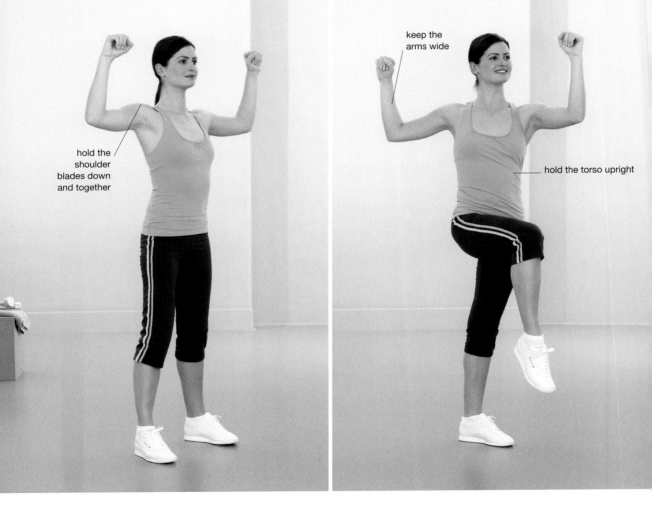

keep the arms wide

hold the shoulder blades down and together

hold the torso upright

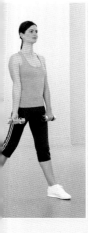

11 Pick up two large free weights. Stand in a staggered lunge position, one foot forward. Hold the weight in your opposite hand, palm forward (see inset). Inhale as you bend your knees into a lunge and bend one elbow to raise the weight to shoulder height. Exhale to return to center. Do 12 reps on each side (1 rep = both sides). **Do your next cardio interval, steps 8–10 (pp. 244–246).**

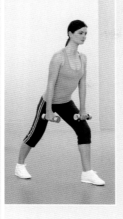

12 Pick up two large free weights and step into a staggered lunge, bending from the hip to 45 degrees (see inset). Inhale as you bend the opposite elbow behind you to 90 degrees, lifting the weight to waist height. Do 12 reps on both sides. **Now do your next cardio interval, steps 8–10 (pp. 244–246).**

keep the elbow close to your side

rest the supporting arm weight on the thigh

press the ball of the foot into the floor

draw the shoulder blades in toward the spine

press the back heel to the floor

>> **squat/triceps kick back**

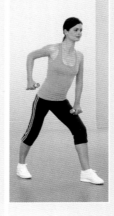

13 Pick up two large free weights and stand with your feet parallel, shoulder width apart, knees soft. Hold the weights palms facing in (see inset). Shift your weight back onto your heels and as you inhale, bend your knees and reach back with your hips. Exhale and return to center, tightening your buttocks as you straighten your legs. Repeat for 12 reps. **Do your next cardio interval, steps 8–10 (pp. 244–246).**

14 Pick up two small free weights and stand in staggered lunge position, one foot back, leaning forward. Bend the elbow on the same side to 90 degrees and raise the upper arm as parallel to the floor as possible (see inset). Breathe in, then exhale as you extend the forearm behind you. Do 12 reps on each side. **Do your next cardio interval, steps 8–10 (pp. 244–246).**

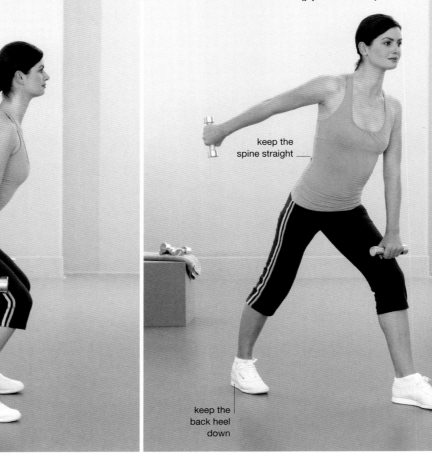

keep the spine straight

reach back with the hips

shift your weight onto the heels

keep the back heel down

>> lat stretch/sun salute

15 To cool down, stand with your feet parallel, hip-width apart, knees soft (see inset). Draw your shoulder blades down and reach both arms up. Interlock your thumbs and center your head between your elbows. Take a few deep breaths to lengthen the spine, lifting the top of your head toward the ceiling, separating your ribs from your hips.

lift the ribs up from the hips

place the feet parallel, hip-width apart

16 Maintaining length in the spine, tighten the hips, thighs, and buttocks. Reach up and out of the low back as you go into a mild back bend. Look up to the ceiling, keeping your head centered between your elbows. Return to center and lower your arms to your sides. Breathe naturally throughout.

look up to the ceiling

lengthen the torso

>> spinal roll-down/plank

17 From the standing position, with your arms by your sides, tuck your chin into your chest and curl down one vertebra at a time. Allow your arms to come forward as you round your spine, feeling your shoulder blades separating. Keep your knees soft. Hold this position, breathing naturally, feeling a stretch in your hamstrings.

18 Walk your hands forward into a plank position, tucking your toes under and planting your wrists under your shoulders. Tighten your abs to keep the lower back from sagging, maintaining a straight line from head to heels. Breathe naturally as you hold the position.

maintain a straight line from head to heels

position the wrists under the shoulders, hands forward

19a

Turn onto your back with knees bent over your hips, calves parallel to the floor, feet relaxed. Be sure to keep a right angle at your knees and hips. Rest your head lightly on your fingertips, thumbs by your ears.

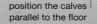

position the calves parallel to the floor

form a 90 degree angle at your hips

19b

Tighten your abs. Inhale, then exhale as you lift your shoulders off the floor, twisting your right shoulder toward your left knee as you extend your right leg. Return to center. Inhale, then exhale as you twist to the other side. Repeat, alternating sides, for 10 reps. (1 rep = both sides).

extend the leg at a 45 degree angle

feel it here

keep the head and shoulders lifted throughout

keep the abs tight

feel it here

>> spinal twist/quad stretch

20 Lie on your back, with both knees bent and your feet on the floor. Stretch your arms out in line with your shoulders, palms down. Drop your knees to one side and turn your head in the opposite direction. Breathe deeply.

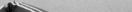

drop the knees to the floor

turn the head in the opposite direction to the knees

21 Turn onto your side, hips and shoulders in line, both knees bent to 45 degrees in front of you. Bend your lower arm and rest your head on it. Reach back with your top arm and draw your foot toward your buttocks, bringing the knee into alignment with your hip. Breathe into the stretch. Repeat the Spinal Twist and Quad Stretch on the other side.

align the knee with the hip

draw the foot toward the buttocks

>> sphinx/child's pose

22 Roll onto your front. Bend your elbows and rest your forearms on the mat. Draw your shoulder blades down as you lift your chest, sliding your elbows forward to be directly under your shoulders. Turn your head to one side, then the other, to stretch the neck. Hold each position and breathe naturally throughout.

feel it here

draw the shoulder blades down and together

press the hips into the floor

feel it here

23 Sit back on your heels and bend forward, forehead reaching to mat, arms stretching center. Walk your hands to one side, keeping your head centered between your elbows, then stretch to the other side. With every exhale, let your body sink deeper into the position.

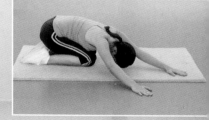

feel it here

position the head centered between the elbows

reach the arms forward

step-touch workout at a glance

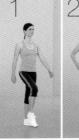
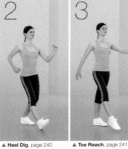
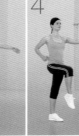
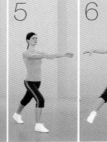
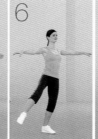
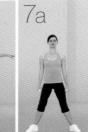
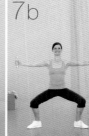

▲ **March,** page 240
▲ **Heel Dig,** page 240
▲ **Toe Reach,** page 241
▲ **Knee Raise,** page 241
▲ **Reverse Lunge,** page 242
▲ **Lateral Lift,** page 242
Repeat Steps 5–1
▲ **Plié with Lateral Raise,** page 243
▲ **Plié with Lateral Raise,** page 243

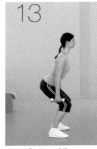
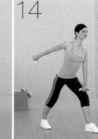
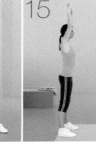
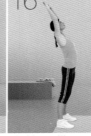
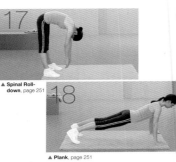

▲ **Squat,** page 249
Repeat Steps 8–10
▲ **Triceps Kick Back,** page 249
Repeat Steps 8–10
▲ **Lat Stretch,** page 250
▲ **Sun Salute,** page 250
▲ **Spinal Roll-down,** page 251
▲ **Plank,** page 251

toning ball workout at a glance

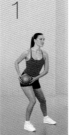
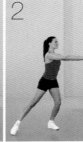
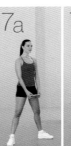
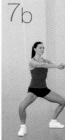
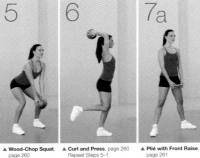

▲ **Rock Lunge,** page 258
▲ **Skater,** page 258
▲ **Pendulum Swing,** page 259
▲ **Body Sway,** page 259
▲ **Wood-Chop Squat,** page 260
▲ **Curl and Press,** page 260
Repeat Steps 5–1
▲ **Plié with Front Raise,** page 261
▲ **Plié with Front Raise,** page 261

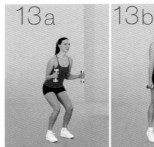

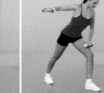
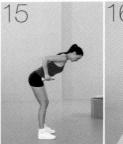
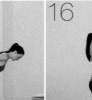

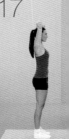

▲ **Squat with Weight Shift,** page 266
▲ **Squat with Weight Shift,** page 266
Repeat Steps 8–10
▲ **Reverse Fly,** page 267
Repeat steps 8–10
▲ **Triceps Kick Back,** page 267
Repeat Steps 8–10
▲ **Lat Stretch,** page 268
▲ **Triceps Stretch,** page 268

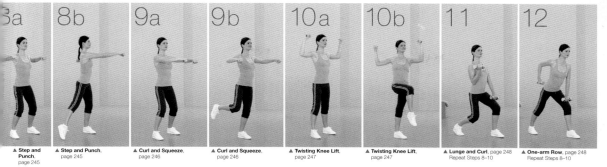

▲ **Step and Punch,** page 245

▲ **Step and Punch,** page 245

▲ **Curl and Squeeze,** page 246

▲ **Curl and Squeeze,** page 246

▲ **Twisting Knee Lift,** page 247

▲ **Twisting Knee Lift,** page 247

▲ **Lunge and Curl,** page 248
Repeat Steps 8–10

▲ **One-arm Row,** page 248
Repeat Steps 8–10

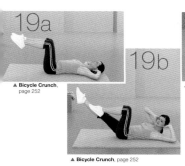

▲ **Bicycle Crunch,** page 252

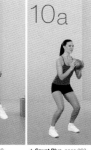

▲ **Bicycle Crunch,** page 252

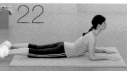

▲ **Spinal Twist,** page 253

▲ **Quad Stretch,** page 253

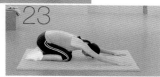

▲ **Sphinx,** page 254

▲ **Child's Pose,** page 254

▲ **Step and Dig,** page 262

▲ **Knee Lift,** page 262

▲ **Squat Plus,** page 263

▲ **Squat Plus,** page 263

▲ **Squat with Knee Lift,** page 264

▲ **Squat with Knee Lift,** page 264
Repeat Steps 8–10

▲ **Lunge and Row,** page 265

▲ **Lunge and Row,** page 265
Repeat Steps 8–10

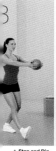

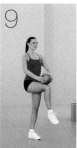

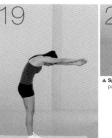

▲ **Side Bend,** page 269

▲ **Forward Bend,** page 269

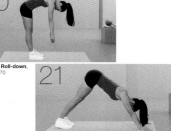

▲ **Spinal Roll-down,** page 270

▲ **Downward Dog,** page 270

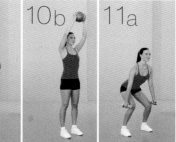

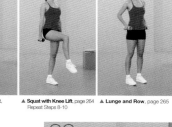

▲ **Plank,** page 271

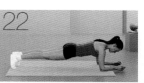

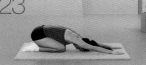

▲ **Child's Pose,** page 271

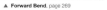

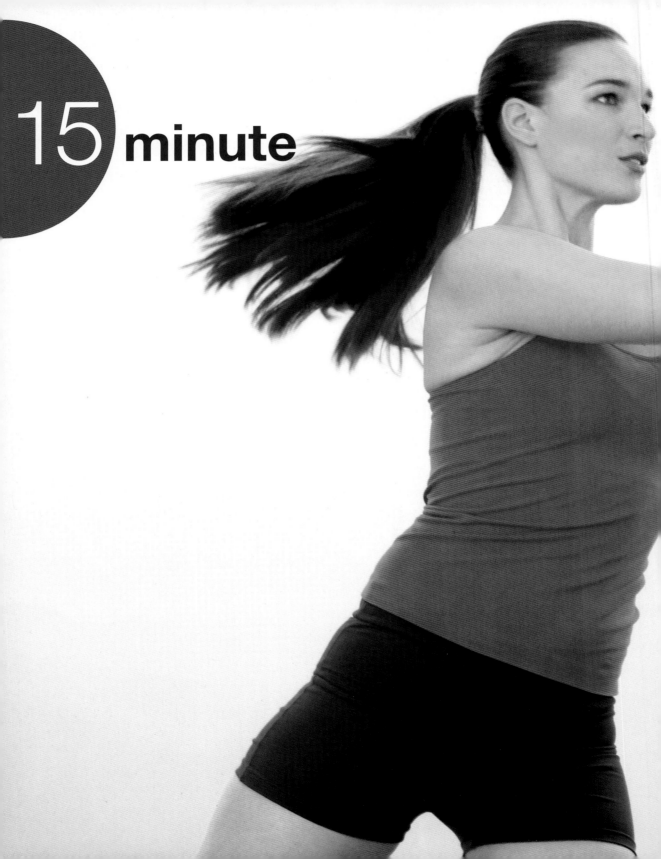

15 minute

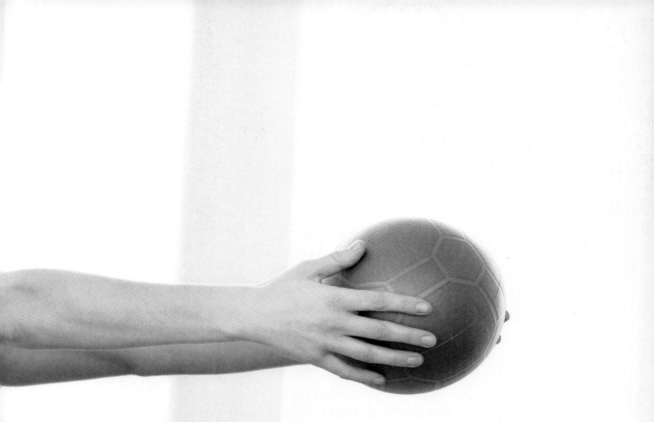

toning ball
workout >>

Improve your coordination
and balance
Add variety to your workout
with a ball

>> **rock lunge/skater**

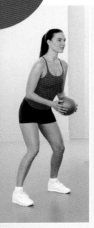

1 To begin your warm up, stand with your feet parallel, slightly wider than shoulder-width apart, knees bent. Lean forward slightly and hold the ball in front of your hips (see inset). Straighten one leg and lunge the other way, moving the ball to your opposite hip. Repeat, alternating sides for a total of 8 reps (1 rep = both sides).

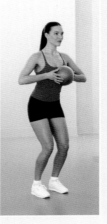

2 Stand with your feet parallel, hip-width apart, knees bent. Hold the ball in front of your chest (see inset). Keep one knee bent and shift your weight onto it as you extend the other leg out to the side, toe resting lightly on the floor. Stretch your arms out diagonally, pressing the ball away from your extended leg. Then return to the starting position and repeat, alternating sides, for a total of 8 reps (1 rep = both sides).

let the head follow the action

press the ball away from the extended leg

move the ball from hip to hip

keep the feet stationary as you lunge

rest the foot lightly on the floor

3 Stand with your feet parallel, shoulder-width apart, knees bent. Hold the ball straight down (see inset). Spring up by extending your arms and legs, sweeping the ball high to one side and lifting the opposite heel. Swing the ball down to the start position, and repeat, alternating sides for 8 reps (1 rep = both sides).

4 Stand with feet parallel, shoulder-width apart, knees slightly bent. Hold the ball overhead (see inset). Step one leg inward and flex at the waist, swinging the ball to the same side. Repeat, alternating sides, for a total of 8 reps (1 rep = both sides).

extend the arms to lift the ball high

twist through the torso

lift the heel off of the floor

draw the shoulder blades down

keep the head centered between the elbows

as you step to the side, touch the feet together

>> wood-chop squat/curl and press

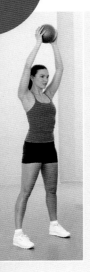

5 Still holding the ball above your head, stand with your feet parallel, shoulder-width apart, knees soft (see inset). Bend your knees into a squat, reaching back with your hips, keeping your heels pressed into the floor. With your arms straight, "chop" the ball down, lowering it to the knees. Repeat 8 times.

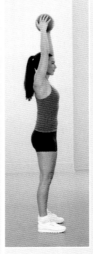

6 Reach the ball toward the ceiling (see inset), then bend both elbows, lowering it behind your head. At the same time, bend one leg back, lifting your heel toward the buttocks. Repeat, alternating legs, for a total of 8 reps (1 rep = both sides). **Repeat Steps 5–1** (reverse order) to complete your warm up.

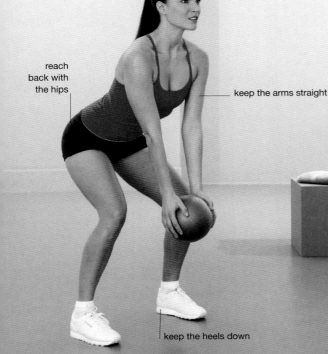

reach back with the hips

keep the arms straight

keep the heels down

maintain a straight line from the elbow to the knee

keep the thighs aligned

>> plié with front raise

7a Put down the ball and pick up one large weight for the first resistance exercise. Stand with your feet slightly wider than shoulder-width apart, shift your weight to your heels, and turn your legs out from the hips until your feet are at 45 degree angles. Hold the weight horizontally with one hand at each end, your arms straight down in front.

7b As you inhale, bend your knees until your thighs are as parallel to the floor as possible; simultaneously lift the weight to shoulder height, keeping your arms straight. Exhale, press through your heels, and tighten your inner and outer thighs as you return to the starting position. Repeat 12 times.

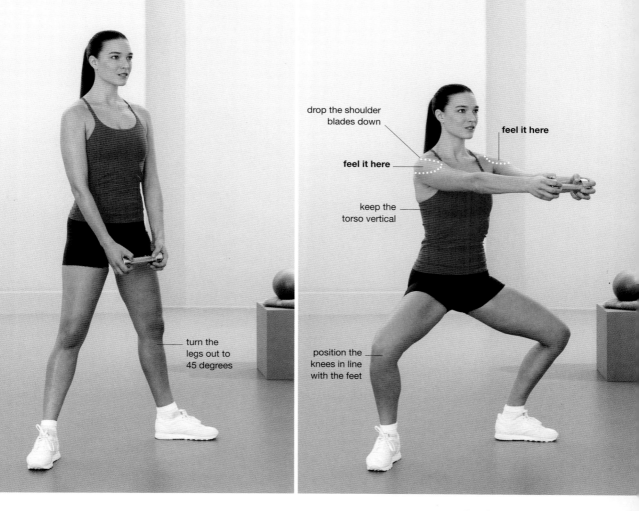

turn the legs out to 45 degrees

drop the shoulder blades down

feel it here

feel it here

keep the torso vertical

position the knees in line with the feet

>> step and dig/knee lift

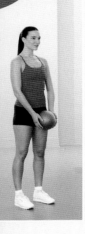

8 Start your first cardio interval. Stand with your feet hip-width apart, knees soft, feet parallel or slightly turned out. Hold the ball with your arms straight down (see inset). Tap your heel to the front, pointing your toes to the ceiling, as you bring the ball up to shoulder height. Keep your arms straight but not stiff. Alternate legs for a total of 8 reps (1 rep = both sides). Breathe naturally throughout.

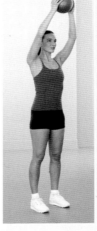

9 Stand with your feet parallel, hip-width apart, knees slightly bent. Hold the ball above your head, with elbows slightly rounded (see inset). Bring your knee up to hip height as you lower the ball toward your knee. Repeat, alternating legs for 8 reps (1 rep = both sides). Breathe naturally throughout.

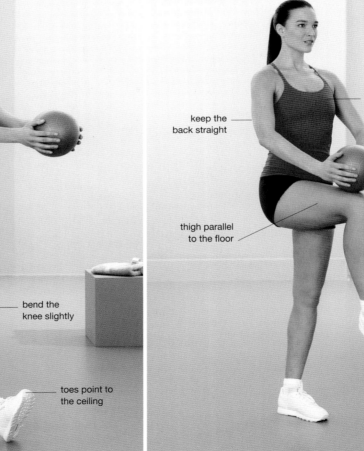

keep the arms straight but not stiff

bend the knee slightly

toes point to the ceiling

keep the back straight

keep the chest lifted

thigh parallel to the floor

>> squat plus

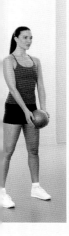

10a Stand with your feet shoulder-width apart, holding the ball with your arms straight down (see inset). Bend your knees into a squat, at the same time bending your elbows to lift the ball to your chest. Keep your weight centered, heels down. Reach back with your hips, keeping your knees behind your toes.

10b Lift the ball up above your head as you straighten your legs. Then bend into the squat, ball to chest (see 10a), before returning to the starting position. Take full, deep breaths. Repeat the sequence 12 times. **Steps 8–10 complete the cardio interval.**

hold the elbows close to the sides

press down through the heels

keep the shoulders down

keep the back straight

straighten the legs

>> squat with knee lift

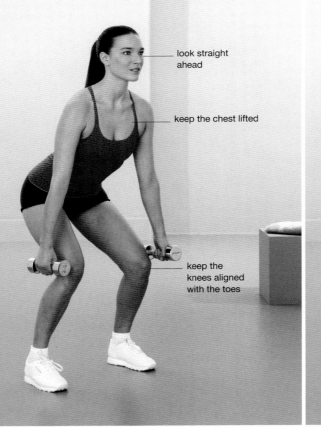

11a Put down the beach ball and pick up two large free weights. Stand with your feet parallel, shoulder-width apart, knees soft. Hold one weight in each hand, with your arms by your sides and palms facing in (see inset). Inhale as you squat: shift your weight back into your heels, reaching back with your hips and letting your torso lean forward. Release your pelvis to allow a natural curve in your back.

11b Exhale and straighten your legs. Shift your weight to one side and bring the other knee up to hip height. Balance for a moment, then return to the starting position (see inset, left). Squat again (see left), straighten your legs, and change sides for the knee lift (see below). Keep your hips level, chest lifted, eyes forward throughout. Repeat for a total of 8 reps (1 rep = both sides). **Do your next cardio interval, steps 8–10 (pp. 262–263).**

look straight ahead

keep the chest lifted

keep the knees aligned with the toes

stand tall

>> **lunge and row**

12a Exchange the ball for two large free weights. Stand with your feet parallel, hip-width apart, knees soft. Hold the weights at your hips, palms in, elbows bent at right angles and close to your sides. Stabilize your shoulder blades by drawing them down and together. Keep your wrists straight, in line with your forearms.

12b Inhale as you step forward with one leg, bending both knees. At the same time, straighten your arms, lowering the weights toward your knee. Exhale as you spring back, pulling the weights to your hips. Alternate legs for 8 reps (1 rep = both sides). **Do the next cardio interval, steps 8–10 (pp. 263–263).**

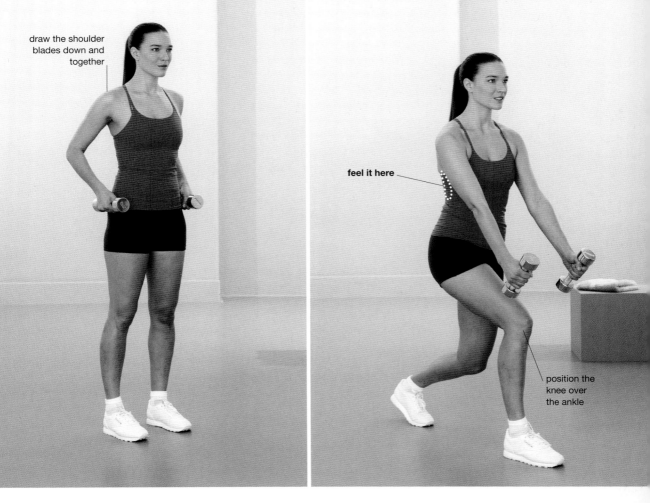

draw the shoulder blades down and together

feel it here

position the knee over the ankle

>> squat with weight shift

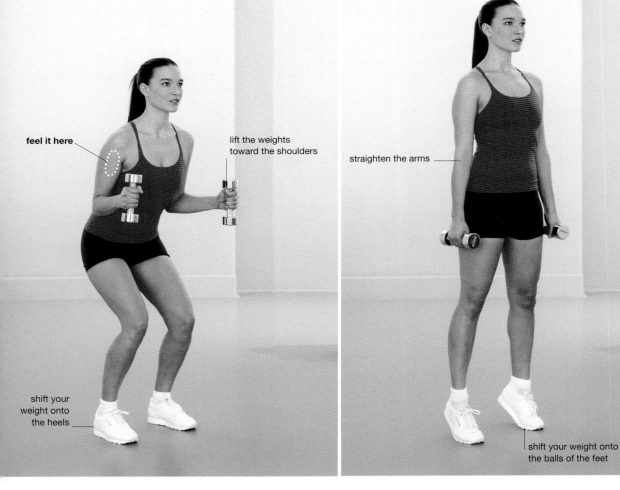

13a Pick up two large weights. Stand with your feet parallel, hip-width apart. Hold the weights by your sides (see inset). Shifting your weight into your heels, inhale as you bend your knees into a squat; at the same time, bend your elbows, bringing the weights up toward your shoulders.

13b Exhale as you straighten your arms and legs to the starting position. Inhale again, then exhale as you shift your weight onto the balls of your feet and lift your heels high. Balance for a moment before lowering the heels onto the floor and preparing for the next squat. Do 8 reps, combining both moves. **Then do your next cardio interval, steps 8–10 (pp. 262–263).**

feel it here

lift the weights toward the shoulders

straighten the arms

shift your weight onto the heels

shift your weight onto the balls of the feet

14 Exchange the ball for two large free weights. Stand in staggered lunge position, one foot forward and the arm on the same side resting on your thigh (see inset). Draw your shoulder blade in and exhale as you lift the other arm out to the side at shoulder height. Repeat 12 times, then switch sides. **Do your next cardio interval, steps 8–10 (pp. 262–263).**

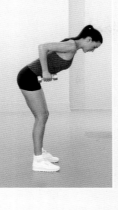

15 Exchange the ball for two large weights. Bend your knees and hinge forward. Bend your elbows to 90 degrees and raise your upper arms parallel to the floor (see inset). Exhale, extending forearms behind. Inhale as you bend your elbows. Repeat 12 times. **Do your next cardio interval, steps 8–10 (pp. 262–263).**

align the head and neck with the spine

feel it here

keep the elbow rounded

feel it here

position the upper arms parallel to the floor

keep the knees slightly bent

>> lat stretch/triceps stretch

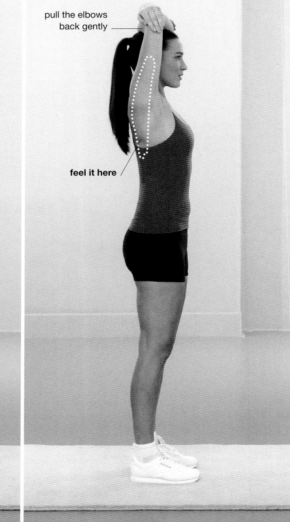

16 Get your mat for the cool down. Stand with your feet parallel, hip-width apart, knees soft. Draw your shoulder blades down (see inset). Reach both arms up above your head, palms facing in. Breathe deeply, separating the vertebrae and lengthening through the spine. Hold the position for two to three breathing cycles.

draw the shoulder blades down

feel it here

stack the ribs over the hips

keep the knees soft

17 Cross your arms and take hold of your elbows. Keep your head centered. Gently pull your elbows back and hold. If this is too difficult, hold one elbow at a time. Use a steady stretch without bouncing to allow the muscle to lengthen gradually. Breathe deeply.

pull the elbows back gently

feel it here

>> side bend/forward bend

18 Still holding your elbows, and with your head centered, lift up from the waist and bend to one side, feeling a stretch all the way down your side to the hip. Hold, breathing into the stretch; then pass through the center and bend to the other side. Hold, take a deep breath and then return to center.

19 From the center position reach forward with your arms at shoulder height. Cross your wrists and turn your palms inward to bring them together, thumbs facing down. Round your upper back, head and neck aligned with your spine, ears between your upper arms. Separate your shoulder blades and reach as far forward as possible. Breathe and relax deeper into the stretch with each exhalation.

keep the head centered between the elbows

allow the shoulder blades to separate

keep the head and neck aligned with the spine

feel it here

keep your weight evenly distributed on the feet

>> **spinal roll-down/downward dog**

20 From the Forward Bend position, drop your arms to your sides, tuck your chin into your chest, and roll down through the spine, one vertebra at a time. Allow your arms to come forward and the shoulder blades to separate.

keep the chin tucked in

keep the knees soft

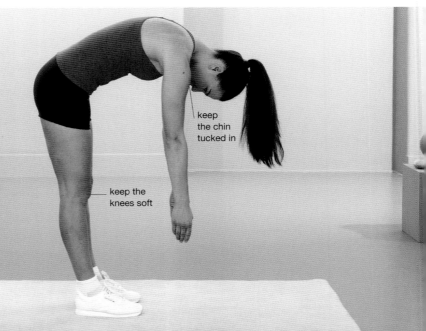

21 Bend down, place your palms on the mat and walk your hands forward. Reach up with your hips and keep lengthening through the spine. Press your heels toward the floor. If necessary, bend your knees slightly to release your lower back. Breathe and stretch.

reach up with the hips

lengthen through the spine

22 Walk forward and place your forearms on the mat, elbows directly under your shoulders, palms facing in, hands in loose fists. Tighten your abdominal and back muscles to keep your torso lifted in a straight line from head to toe. Tuck your toes under slightly: you will feel a stretch in your calves. Hold the position, breathing naturally.

keep the shoulder blades down

23 Bend your knees and reach back with your hips until your buttocks rest on your heels. At the same time round forward, curving the spine, forehead toward floor. Reach your arms to the front to stretch your lats, chest, and shoulders. With every exhale, sink deeper into the position; mind and body calm. Move back into the plank, bending your elbows and straightening your legs. Finally, repeat the Child's Pose to complete your cool down.

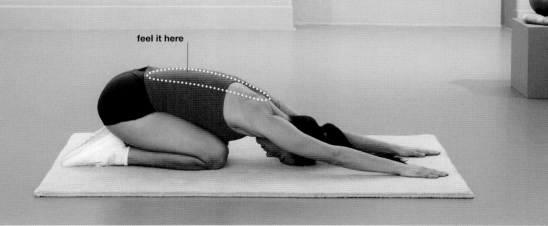

feel it here

15 minute

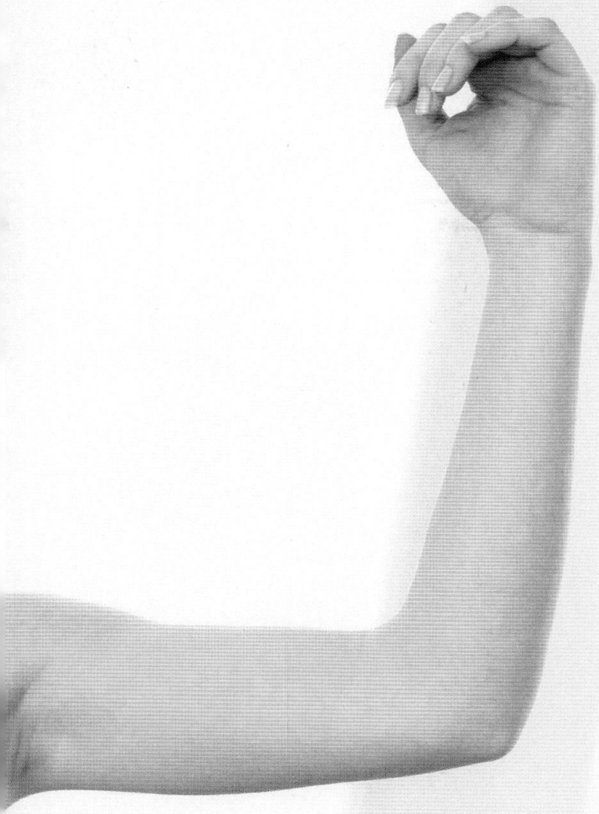

hop, jig, and jump
workout >>

Experience the childlike joy
of hopping and jumping
Release endorphins with this
upbeat workout

>> bend and raise/double arm swing

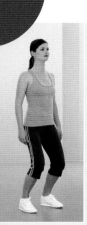

1 To warm up, stand with your feet parallel, hip-width apart, knees soft, arms by your sides. Tighten your abs and lift your chest. Bend your knees (see inset) then straighten your legs. Shift your weight to the balls of your feet and lift your heels, resisting the floor. Continue bending and then rising up, allowing your arms to swing naturally forward, for a total of 8 times.

2 Continue to bend your knees rhythmically as you swing your arms to back and front. From the starting position of bent knees (see inset, left), feet flat on the floor, straighten your legs and swing your arms behind. Bend your knees again as your arms pass through the center and then swing them in front as you straighten your legs. Repeat for a total of 8 swings, back to front.

look straight ahead

shift your weight to the balls of the feet

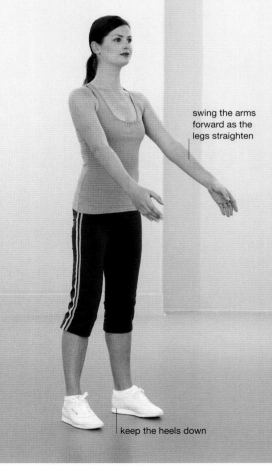

swing the arms forward as the legs straighten

keep the heels down

>> **single arm swing/cross and open**

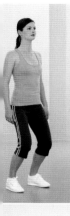

3 Continue to bend your knees rhythmically (see inset), but change the arms, swinging one forward and the other back every time you straighten your legs. Keep your heels down, knees in line with toes. Keep your shoulder blades down as you swing your arms. Your chest stays lifted, chin level. Repeat, alternating arms, for a total of 8 reps (1 rep = both sides).

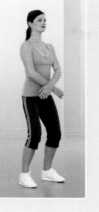

4 Continuing with rhythmic knee bends, change your arms to cross in front as you bend your knees (see inset) and then lift them out to the sides as you straighten your legs. Keep your shoulder blades down as you lift your arms to shoulder height, palms down. Bend and straighten, lifting your arms out to the sides, 16 times.

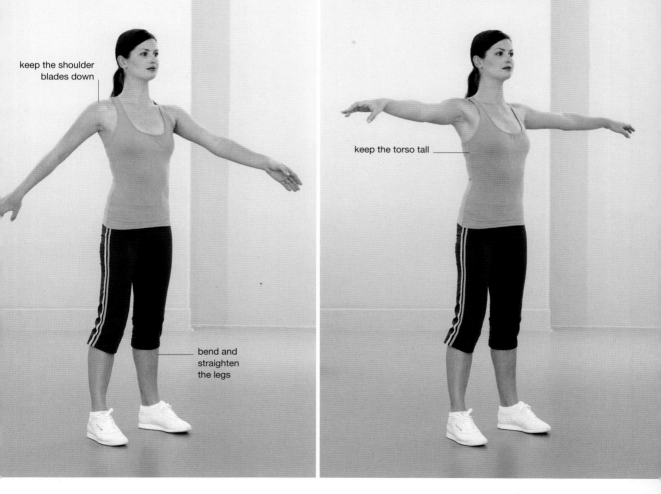

keep the shoulder blades down

bend and straighten the legs

keep the torso tall

>> **lateral lift/jumping jack**

5 Arms stay the same as you bend and straighten your knees, but you add a side leg lift. Bend your knees as you cross your arms in front (see inset), then straighten both legs and lift one to the side as you raise your arms. Keep your hips level, shoulders down. Repeat, alternating legs, for a total of 8 reps (1 rep = both sides).

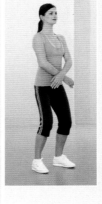

6 Continue to raise and lower your arms, but change your legs. As you cross your arms in front (see inset), jump your feet together. As you raise your arms to shoulder height, tap one foot out to the side. Alternate sides for 8 reps (1 rep = both sides). **Repeat Steps 5–1** (reverse order) to complete your warm up.

lift the arms to shoulder height

lift the leg to the side

bend and straighten the legs

tap the toe out to the side

>> hip hinge and reverse fly

7a
Pick up two small weights for your first resistance exercise. Stand up straight, feet parallel, hip-width apart, shoulders down. Hold a weight in each hand in front of your thighs, palms facing back (see inset). Bend your knees as you hinge forward from the hips, maintaining neutral spine alignment. The weights are now directly under your shoulders.

7b
Inhale, then, as you exhale, raise your arms to the sides, in line with the shoulders, to shoulder height. Keep shoulder blades together as you lift your arms, elbows rounded, palms backward. Inhale and lower your arms, then exhale as you straighten your hips and knees to return to start position (see inset, left). Repeat combination for 8 reps.

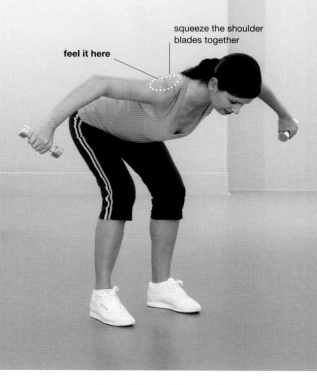

keep the spine straight, parallel to the floor

hold the weights directly under the shoulders

feel it here

squeeze the shoulder blades together

>> step-hop/jig

8 Put down the weights for the first cardio interval. Stand with your feet parallel, hip-width apart, arms by your sides. Step forward with one leg and hop on it, as your raise the other knee to hip height. The arm opposite the raised leg swings forward, elbow bent. Lower the leg and step back to the starting position. Alternate legs, swinging your arms in opposition, for a total of 6 reps (1 rep = both sides).

9 To begin, jump in place, feet hip width apart, hands on your hips. Hop on one leg, extending the other leg on a diagonal, digging your heel into the floor, toe pointing toward the ceiling. Bring the exended leg back and repeat on the other side. Keep your upper body vertical, chest lifted, eyes looking straight ahead. Alternate legs for a total of 8 reps (1 rep = both sides).

keep the arms close to the sides

step forward and hop

10 With your feet together, arms out to the sides, contract your abs and jump up, rotating your hips to one side. Turn your hips, knees, and feet as a unit. Land with your knees bent. Keep your torso upright, your shoulders facing forward. Alternate sides for a total of 8 reps (1 rep = both sides). **Steps 8–10 complete your cardio interval, which you will repeat after each resistance exercise.**

11a Pick up one large free weight. Step forward with one leg into a staggered lunge position. Hold the weight with both hands horizontally in front of your waist, elbows bent. Keep your weight centered between your legs, your back heel down and your feet parallel. Your shoulders should be square to the front, your eyes looking straight ahead.

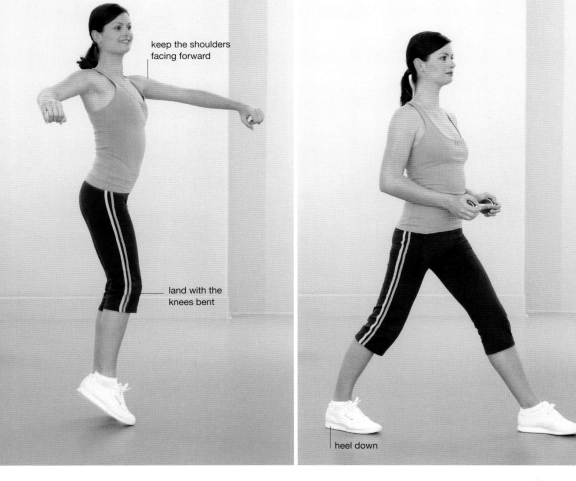

keep the shoulders facing forward

land with the knees bent

heel down

>> lunge and twist

11b Inhale as you bend both knees into a low lunge. Bend your front knee at a right angle directly over the ankle, the thigh parallel to the floor; bend your back knee close to the floor with the back heel lifted. As you come into the lunge, twist through your torso, reaching the weight toward your little toe. Keep your shoulder blades drawn together and your head and neck aligned with your spine, being careful not to round the upper back.

11c Exhale as you return to the starting position and then lift the weight high on a diagonal above your opposite shoulder, elbows bent. Keep looking forward. Do 6 reps of the sequence, bending your knees into a lunge as you lower the weight before lifting it again. Switch sides for another 6 reps. **Then do your next cardio interval, steps 8–10 (pp. 278–279).**

twist through the torso

feel it here

keep the spine straight

lift the heel up

>> side-squat jump

12a Stand with your feet parallel, hip-width apart, knees soft, your hands on your hips. Step one leg to the side so that your feet are shoulder-width apart (see inset). Shift your weight back onto your heels as you bend your knees into a squat. Reach back with your hips, keeping your chest lifted.

12b Spring from both feet, jumping straight up. Land in a squat, knees bent, weight centered. Straighten your legs, step back to center, and repeat, stepping to the other side. Do 4 reps (1 rep = both sides) for a total of 8 squats. **Do the next cardio interval, steps 8–10 (pp. 278–279).**

keep the chest lifted

step to the side before squatting

jump several inches off the floor

>> balance and press/plié and curl

13 Stand with feet parallel, hip-width apart. Hold two small weights at shoulder height (see inset). Exhale, extending one arm, lifting opposite knee. Balance, inhale and step in place, alternating sides for 8 reps (1 rep = both sides). **Do your next cardio interval, steps 8–10 (pp. 278–279).**

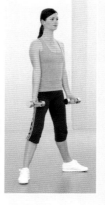

14 Pick up two large weights, holding one in each hand. Stand in a wide stance, legs turned out to 45 degrees. Keep your arms by your sides (see inset). Inhale and bend your knees and elbows at the same time, lifting the weights toward your shoulders. Exhale as you straighten your arms and legs. **Do your next cardio interval, steps 8–10 (pp. 278–279).**

keep the palms facing in

lengthen through the spine to maintain balance

feel it here

hold the elbows close to your sides

15a Pick up two small weights. Stand with your feet parallel, hip-width apart, knees bent. Hold one weight in each hand, arms by your sides, palms facing inward. Make sure your torso is aligned and ready for action: stack your ribs over your hips, engage the abs, draw your shoulder blades down, and lift your chest.

15b Inhale, then exhale as you straighten your legs, lifting one to the side, as you raise both arms to shoulder height, palms down. Your arms should be straight but not stiff. Inhale, then return to the starting position, bending the knees and squaring the hips. Alternate legs, lifting both arms every time for 12 reps (1 rep = both sides).

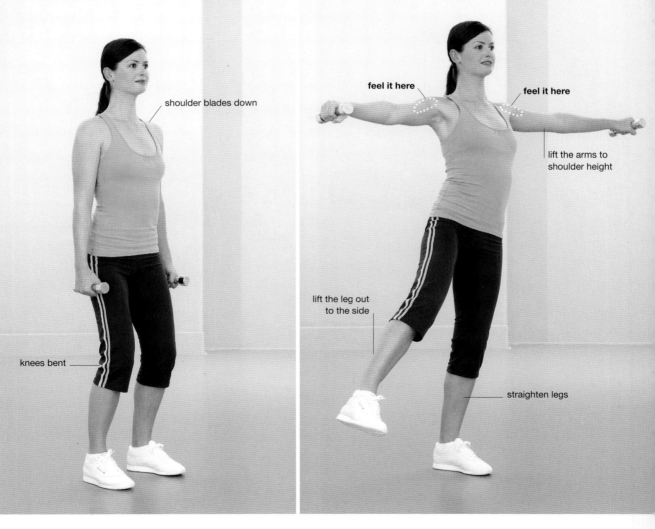

shoulder blades down

feel it here

feel it here

lift the arms to shoulder height

lift the leg out to the side

knees bent

straighten legs

>> flat back stretch/spinal twist

16 Get your mat for the cool down, and stand with your legs hip-width apart, hands on your hips. Lengthen through your spine, lifting the top of your head toward the ceiling. Draw your shoulder blades down and together. Bend forward from your hips until your back is parallel to the floor, still elongating the spine by reaching your head forward. Keep your knees straight, but not locked. Breathe deeply while you hold the stretch.

17 From the flat back position, reach one hand across your body to the opposite foot, and lift the other arm straight up to the ceiling, palm forward. If you are able, press the heel of your supporting hand down on the mat. However, you may be more comfortable resting it on your ankle. Keep your knees straight and your hips level. Breathe naturally throughout, then switch sides and repeat.

feel it here

keep the legs straight but not stiff

keep the hips level

feel it here

feel it here

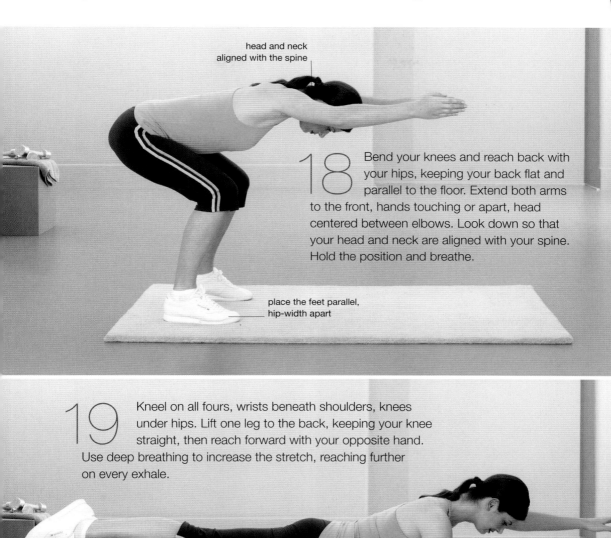

head and neck
aligned with the spine

18 Bend your knees and reach back with your hips, keeping your back flat and parallel to the floor. Extend both arms to the front, hands touching or apart, head centered between elbows. Look down so that your head and neck are aligned with your spine. Hold the position and breathe.

place the feet parallel,
hip-width apart

19 Kneel on all fours, wrists beneath shoulders, knees under hips. Lift one leg to the back, keeping your knee straight, then reach forward with your opposite hand. Use deep breathing to increase the stretch, reaching further on every exhale.

hold the leg
at hip height

>> calf stretch/spinal curve

20

Keep your arms planted and extend one leg behind you, placing your toes on the floor and pressing the heel back. Breathe naturally as you stretch, then switch legs.

feel it here

press the heel back

21

Kneel on all fours, knees under your hips, hip-width apart. Position your wrists under your shoulders. Lift your head and your hips up, curving the spine into a "C" shape. Alternate this with the Spinal Arch on the opposite page, repeating 3 times in all.

lift the head up

feel it here

lift the hips up

22
Start from a kneeling positon, knees under hips, wrists under shoulders, your back neutral. Then arch your spine, rounding it up to the ceiling by tucking your hips under and dropping your head between your arms. Alternate this with Spinal Curve (see 21, opposite), repeating 3 times in all.

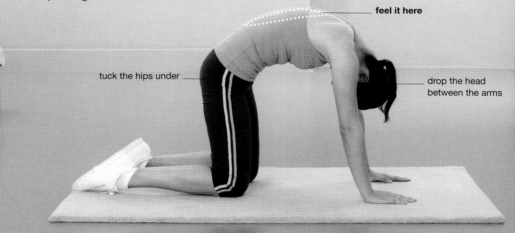

feel it here

tuck the hips under

drop the head between the arms

23
Sit back, reaching your hips toward your heels, at the same time rounding forward and extending your arms in front of you until your head rests on the mat. Keep your elbows off the mat to get the best stretch. Sink down into the position, holding for 3 deep breathing cycles, and sinking deeper into the position with each exhalation to complete your cool down.

feel it here

reach the hips toward the heels

hop, jig, and jump workout at a glance

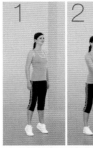 1
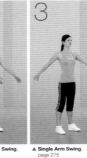 2
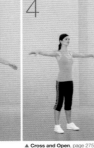 3
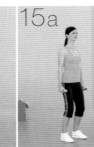 4
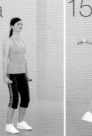 5
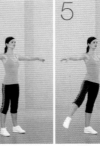 6
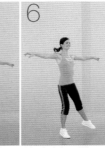 7a
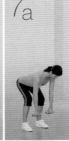 7b
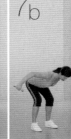

▲ **Bend and Raise,** page 274

▲ **Double Arm Swing,** page 274

▲ **Single Arm Swing,** page 275

▲ **Cross and Open,** page 275

▲ **Lateral Lift,** page 276

▲ **Jumping Jack,** page 276 Repeat Steps 5–1

▲ **Hip Hinge and Reverse Fly,** page 277

▲ **Hip Hinge and Reverse Fly,** page 277

13
14
15a
15b
16
17

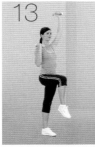
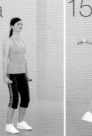
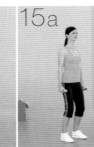
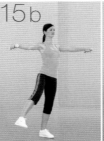

▲ **Balance and Press,** page 282 Repeat Steps 8–10

▲ **Plié and Curl,** page 282 Repeat Steps 8–10

▲ **Lateral Lift,** page 283

▲ **Lateral Lift,** page 283

▲ **Flat Back Stretch,** page 284

▲ **Spinal Twist,** page 284

lunge around the clock workout at a glance

1
2
3
4
5a
5b
6
7

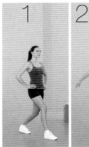
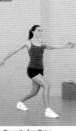
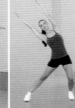
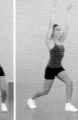
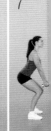

▲ **Front Lunge,** page 292

▲ **Opposite Arm Raise,** page 292

▲ **Arm Reach,** page 293

▲ **Diagonal Lunge,** page 293

▲ **Side Lunge,** page 294

▲ **Side Lunge,** page 294

▲ **Reverse Lunge,** page 295 Repeat Steps 5–1

▲ **Wood-Chop Squat,** page 295

13a
13b
14a
14b
15
16

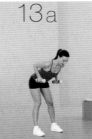
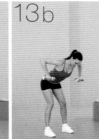
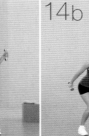
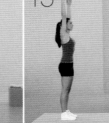

▲ **Bent-Over Row,** page 300

▲ **Bent-Over Row,** page 300 Repeat steps 8–10

▲ **Lift and Squat,** page 301

▲ **Lift and Squat,** page 301 Repeat Steps 8–10

▲ **Upper Body Stretch,** page 302

▲ **Downward Dog,** page 302

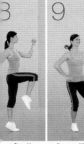
▲ **Step-Hop,** page 278

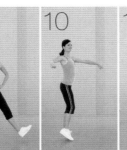
▲ **Jig,** page 278

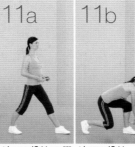
▲ **Jump and Twist,** page 279

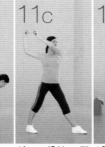
▲ **Lunge and Twist,** page 279

▲ **Lunge and Twist,** page 280

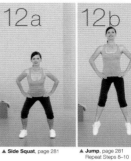
▲ **Lunge and Twist,** page 280 Repeat Steps 8–10

▲ **Side Squat,** page 281

▲ **Jump,** page 281 Repeat Steps 8–10

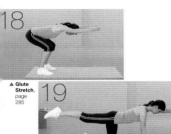
▲ **Glute Stretch,** page 285

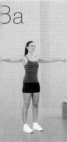
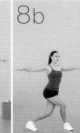
▲ **Arm and Leg Lift,** page 285

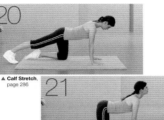
▲ **Calf Stretch,** page 286

▲ **Spinal Curve,** page 286

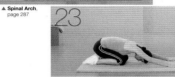
▲ **Spinal Arch,** page 287

▲ **Child's Pose,** page 287

▲ **Curtsy Lunge,** page 296

▲ **Curtsy Lunge,** page 296

▲ **Charleston Lunge,** page 297

▲ **Charleston Lunge,** page 297

▲ **Push-off Lunge,** page 298

▲ **Push-off Lunge,** page 298

▲ **Plié and Row,** page 299 Repeat Steps 8–10

▲ **Balance Squat,** page 299 Repeat Steps 8–10

▲ **Half Push-up and Side Plank,** page 303

▲ **Half Push-up and Side Plank,** page 303

▲ **Child's Pose,** page 304

▲ **Kneeling Lunge,** page 304

▲ **Cross-Legged Stretch,** page 305

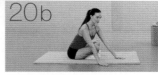
▲ **Cross-Legged Stretch,** page 305

15 minute

lunge around the clock >>

Challenge yourself with
more complex moves
Advance your skills
and fitness levels

>> **front lunge/opposite arm raise**

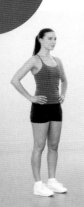

1 To warm up, stand with feet parallel, hip-width apart, knees soft, hands on hips (see inset). Inhale as you step forward, bending knees slightly. Then exhale and push off with your front leg to spring back to the center. Alternate sides for 8 reps (1 rep = both sides).

2 Continue to lunge, alternating legs, and add your arms. From the starting position, feet parallel, hip-width apart, step forward, bending your knees a little deeper, lifting your back heel and always keeping your knee over the ankle. At the same time, raise your hands to shoulder height, palms in, the opposite arm to the front and the other one behind. Keep your torso upright, chest lifted, chin level. Alternate legs and arms for 8 reps (1 rep = both sides).

bend the knees slightly

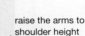

raise the arms to shoulder height

bend the knees a little deeper

>> arm reach/diagonal lunge

3 Continue to lunge, but now raise both arms to the front, lifting as you lunge, and increasing the bend in your knees. Pull your shoulder blades down and together to stabilize them as you extend your arms forward. Lower your arms to your sides as you return to center. Continue, alternating legs, for 8 reps (1 rep = both sides).

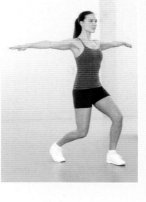

4 From the center, pivot on the back foot and step out to 11 o'clock, lifting your arms to the sides (see inset). Spring back to center, lowering your arms, then lunge out on the opposite diagonal to 1 o'clock. Repeat for 8 reps.

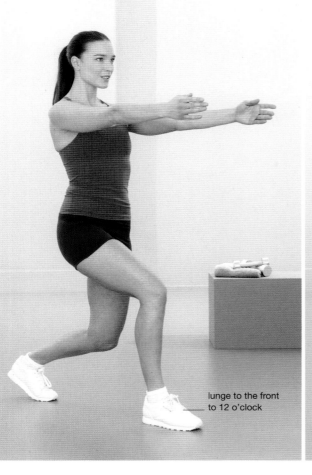

lunge to the front to 12 o'clock

step the front foot out on a diagonal to 1 o'clock

>> **side lunge**

5a Stand with your feet parallel, hip-width apart. Raise your arms to the sides at shoulder height, palms down. Keep your abs tight, hips square to the front, chest lifted. Draw your shoulder blades down and together as you prepare to lunge.

5b Inhale and step your left leg out to the side (9 o'clock), bending your knee. At the same time reach your arms high, turning the palms in, and flex your torso toward the center, bending sideways at the waist. Exhale and spring back to center, rotating the palms down as you lower your arms to shoulder height. Alternate sides (lunge to 3 o'clock) for 8 reps (1 rep = both sides).

keep the leg straight

lunge to the side to 9 o'clock

6 Start in the center position, feet parallel, arms by your sides (see inset). Inhale as you lunge to the back (6 o'clock), landing on the ball of your foot, and bending both knees. At the same time, reach both arms high in front, palms in. Exhale and return to center, arms by your sides. Repeat for 8 reps (1 rep = both sides). **Repeat Steps 5–1** (reverse order) to complete your warm up.

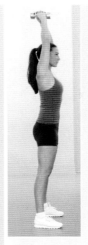

7 Pick up one large weight. Standing with your feet parallel, shoulder width apart, hold the weight overhead (see inset). Inhale as you squat, lowering the weight to your knees as if you are chopping wood. Exhale as you return to the starting position and repeat for 12 reps.

lunge back to 6 o'clock

feel it here

keep the chest lifted

keep the knees behind the toes

>> **curtsy lunge**

8a Put down the weight for your first cardio interval. Stand with your feet parallel, hip-width apart, knees soft. Raise your arms out to the sides at shoulder height, palms down. Keep your elbows slightly rounded. Stand tall, lengthening through your spine by lifting the top of your head toward the ceiling and engaging the abs.

8b Step back on a diagonal, landing on the ball of your foot, heel lifted. Bend both knees and squeeze your shoulder blades together every time you curtsy. Keep your arms at shoulder height. Breathe naturally throughout. Repeat for 8 reps, alternating legs (1 rep = both sides).

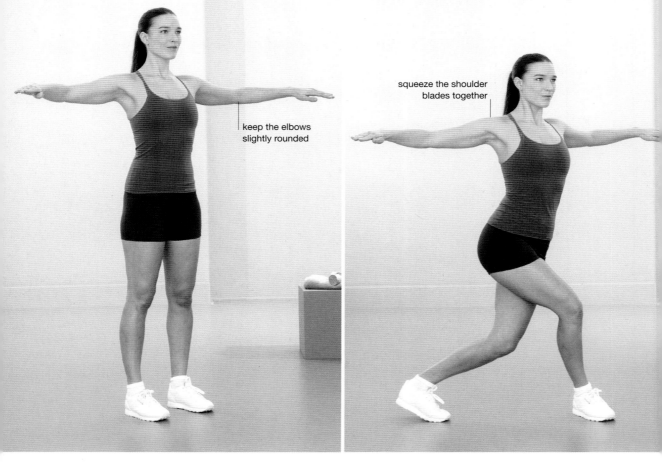

keep the elbows slightly rounded

squeeze the shoulder blades together

>> charleston lunge

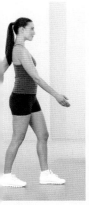

9a Step forward with the lead leg (see inset) and kick the other leg in front of you, knee to hip height. Then swing the leg back and step in place. Swing your arms in opposition to your legs. Continue the movement with the Reverse Lunge (see 9b).

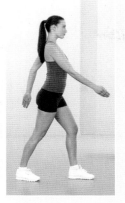

9b Reverse lunge with the lead leg (see inset). Continue a series of step, kick front (see 9a), step, lunge back. Switch arms with every leg change. Repeat 6 times. Change legs by substituting the last lunge with a step in place. Repeat the sequence 6 times on the other side.

swing the arms in opposition to the legs

lunge back with the lead leg

>> push-off lunge

10a Start from a staggered lunge position, your front knee over your ankle. Your back heel should lift easily. Reach your arms overhead on a diagonal, palms in. Center your weight between your legs, torso square to the front, eyes looking forward. Prepare to push off with your back foot.

10b Push off with your back foot, shifting your weight to your front leg, and pump your knee to hip height. At the same time, bend your arms, pulling your elbows to your sides, hands to hip level. Balance for a moment on the supporting leg before lunging again. Repeat a total of 8 times, then change to the other side. Breathe naturally throughout. **You have now completed the cardio interval, which you will repeat after each resistance exercise.**

reach the arms up on a diagonal

keep the knee directly over the ankle

prepare to push off

keep the elbows bent close to the sides

lift the knee to hip height

>> plié and row/balance squat

11 Pick up two small weights. Stand with your legs turned out, slightly wider than shoulder-width apart. Hold a weight in each hand, arms straight down, palms facing back (see inset). Inhale as you bend your knees over your toes and pull the weights to your chest, elbows bending out to the sides. Exhale and straighten up, lowering the weights. Move up and down 12 times. **Do your next cardio interval, steps 8–10 (pp. 296–298).**

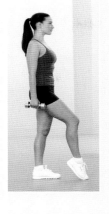

12 Stand with all your weight on one leg, the other leg resting lightly to the front (see inset). Inhale, reach back with your hips and squat on the working leg. Exhale up. Repeat 12 times, then change sides. **Do your next cardio interval, steps 8–10 (pp. 296–298).**

feel it here

feel it here

keep the elbows below shoulder level

turn the legs out at the hips

place the feet at 45 degree angles

keep the torso upright or leaning slightly forward

rest the front leg lightly for balance

>> **bent-over row**

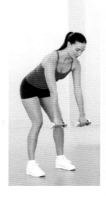

13a Pick up two weights. Stand with your feet parallel, shoulder-width apart, holding a weight in each hand, arms by your sides, palms in. Bend your knees and hinge forward from the hips, keeping your spine in neutral alignment (see inset). Draw your shoulder blades together and exhale as you lift the weights, bending your elbows until the upper arms are parallel to the floor.

13b Lower the weights to the starting position and rotate your arms so that your palms face back (see inset). Pull your shoulder blades together and exhale as you bend your elbows out to the sides until your upper arms are parallel to the floor. Do 8 reps, alternating the position of the arms. **Do your next cardio interval, steps 8–10 (pp. 296–298).**

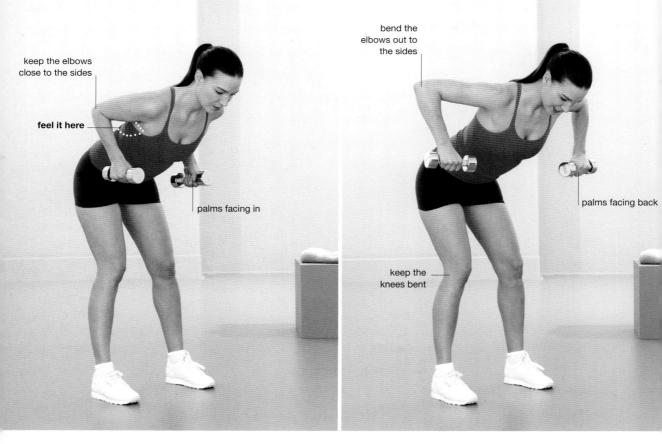

keep the elbows close to the sides

feel it here

palms facing in

bend the elbows out to the sides

palms facing back

keep the knees bent

>> **lift and squat**

14a Pick up two small weights. Stand feet parallel, shoulder-width apart. Hold a weight in each hand, arms by your sides (see inset). Shift your weight to the balls of your feet and lift the heels high; at the same time, bend your elbows, lifting the weights toward your shoulders. Balance, then return to the starting position.

14b Plant your heels on the floor, shift your weight back, and bend your knees into a squat. At the same time, raise your arms behind you, elbows straight. Straighten up, then repeat the combination of rising onto the balls of the feet followed by squatting for 8 reps. Breathe naturally throughout. **Do your next cardio interval, steps 8–10 (pp. 296–298).**

hold the elbows close to the sides

feel it here

keep the elbows straight and close to the sides

lift the heels high

shift your weight to the balls of the feet

shift your weight onto the heels

>> **upper body stretch/downward dog**

15 Get your mat for the cool down. Standing, clasp your hands behind you (see inset) and lift them toward the ceiling. Then bring your arms up, palms in, and reach high. Clasp your wrist and pull to one side, stretching down to your hip; change sides and pull the other way.

feel it here

keep the shoulder blades down

breathe deeply throughout

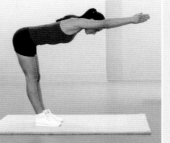

16 Return to center and hinge forward from the hip; knees and back straight. Reach back with the hips as you extend the arms forward, lengthening the spine (see inset). Hold the stretch and breathe. Bend down, place your palms on the mat, and walk your hands forward into Downward Dog, reaching your hips toward the ceiling and pressing your heels toward the mat. If necessary, bend your knees to release the hips and heels. Keep the breath flowing.

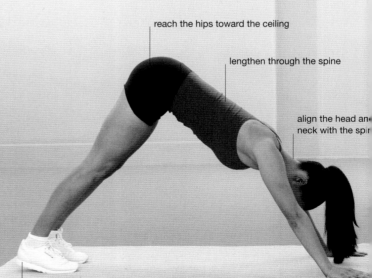

reach the hips toward the ceiling

lengthen through the spine

align the head and neck with the spine

press the heels toward the mat

>> half push-up and side plank

17a

Kneel with your wrists under your shoulders, 3–4 inches (7.5–10 cm) wider than shoulder-width apart (see inset). Drop your hips and shift your weight forward so there is no direct pressure on the kneecaps. Inhale, bend your elbows out to the sides and lower your chest toward the mat. Exhale and push up.

pull the abs tight

17b

Turn onto your side, knees and lower legs stacked, hips and ribs lifted, a straight line from shoulder to knees. The supporting arm is straight, wrist directly under the shoulder. Reach your top arm to the ceiling, palm forward. Repeat the Half Push-up (see 17a) and then do a Side Plank to the other side, alternating for 3 sets (1 set = Push-up, Side Plank, Push-up, Side Plank).

reach the top arm to the ceiling

place the supporting arm under the shoulder

stack the knees and the lower legs

>> child's pose/kneeling lunge

18 Come onto your knees and sit back, reaching your hips toward your heels. At the same time, round forward and reach your arms to the front, forehead to mat. Allow your body to relax and sink into the position.

feel it here

19 Come up onto one knee, bending the other one in front of you, foot on the mat. Raise your arms overhead, palms in, head centered between your elbows. Press your hips forward until you feel a stretch in the front of your hip, the hip flexor. Breathe into the stretch and hold. Then sit back into Child's Pose (see step 18). Repeat the lunge on the other side.

keep the hips square to the front

20a Sit back on your buttocks and cross your legs comfortably in front. Bend forward from the hips with your back straight, keep the sitbones anchored on the floor, and extend your arms to the front. Breathe deeply and relax into the position.

keep the back straight ____

keep the sitbones ____
anchored

20b To finish cooling down, walk your hands to one side, turning your torso to face that knee. Hold the position briefly and breathe deeply, trying to relax more deeply into the position with each exhalation. Pass through center and repeat on the other side. Remember to keep your sitbones anchored throughout.

position the torso
to face the knee ____

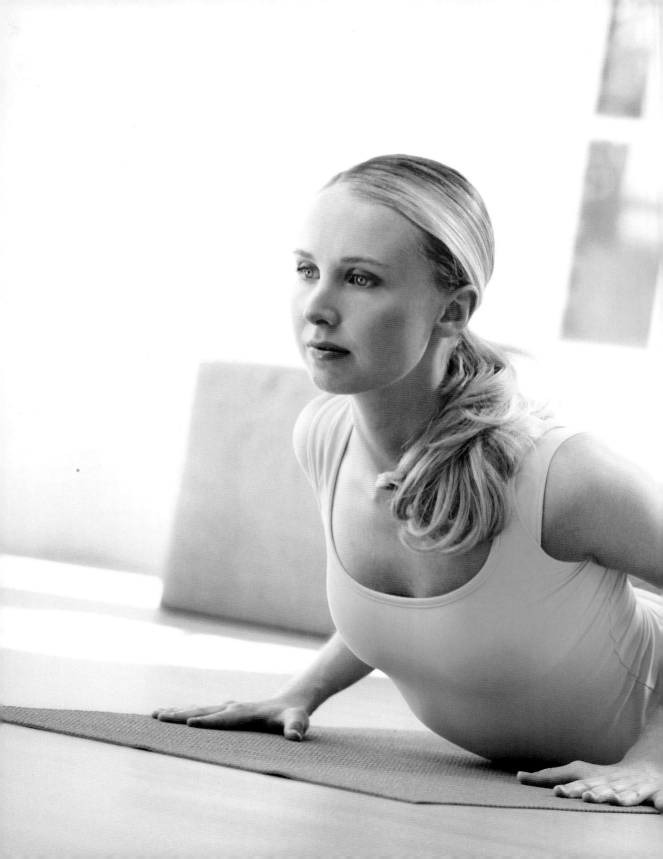

gentle
yoga

Louise Grime

>> yoga for everyone

Welcome to yoga, whether you are trying it out to feel more fit and more flexible, or to de-stress and energize your mind and body. As you practice, you may find that yoga becomes a way of life and you start to approach every aspect of your day with an inquiring, balanced yoga mind-set.

When you embrace yoga, it becomes much more than what you do on the mat—it begins to filter into your way of thinking and interacting with others. As the postures and breathing practices make you feel bright and alive, so your self-confidence and energy levels soar; as you begin to notice where in the body you hold tension, and free it up by stretching and breathing more effectively, so you begin to become less stressed in your mind, too, and more able to appreciate life from different perspectives— just as yoga postures ask you to see the world upside down, backward, or sideways. As your physical balance improves, so does your ability to adopt a more measured approach to decision making and problem solving, enhancing every aspect of life, from your relationships at home and work to the way in which you do business. Above all, yoking together your body and mind with the single focus of a yoga posture makes every part of you feel more harmonious.

What is hatha yoga?

In the West, we tend to think of yoga as a system of physical exercises (known as *asanas*) and breathing techniques (known as *pranayama*). But this type of yoga—*hatha* yoga—is simply one route toward the ultimate aim of yoga, which is to feel so profoundly at peace within that we become aware of a connection with everything else in the universe. In India, where yoga originated many thousands of years ago, people follow other yoga paths to the same end-state of harmonious union:

> ## >> weaving yoga into your life
>
> - **Try to joyfully accept** your current physical limitations. Learn to work with stiff hamstrings or tight shoulders, rather than struggle against them, and you'll become more adept more quickly.
>
> - **Don't be dispirited** when you first begin yoga. Keep a sense of humor, and be kind to your body, and the knots in your mind will also start to unwind.
>
> - **Be patient and watch your breath** rather than pushing yourself to compete, and soon you will experience the bliss of yoga.

bhakti yoga, the path of religious worship; *karma* yoga, doing selfless service for others (Mother Teresa epitomizes this path of yoga); *jnana* yoga, studying yogic philosophy; and *raja* yoga, meditation. Each of these yoga paths suits a different personality type. You have probably turned to *hatha* yoga, the physical aspect of yoga, because, like many of us in the West, you are interested in boosting your health and well-being, and would like to achieve a little more inner peace. As you clean and loosen out your body with its postures, you taste the lightness of being that is *hatha* yoga.

Finding a teacher

When you practice yoga with a teacher, you gain expert advice, as well as invaluable hands-on adjustments. Working with a teacher also helps you gain the confidence to progress to more difficult poses and to work with breathing and meditation techniques. If you attend a regular yoga class, you will also build up a network of supportive fellow students to help you maintain motivation.

But how do you find a teacher to suit you, and a style of yoga from the many confusing options on offer? The best way is to visit a yoga center or gym close to your home or workplace. You can also look for local classes on notice boards in your doctors' office and library, for example. Ask for a list of classes and a description of the style of class if it is not a general "hatha yoga" class (which may draw on a mix of styles—*hatha* yoga can be taught in myriad ways). Iyengar yoga, the most practiced form of yoga across the globe, focuses on alignment and precision in the physical postures using props such as blocks and belts, and offers a sound foundation for beginners. If you enjoy fast-moving exercise, you might try *Ashtanga vinyasa* classes, which teach a seamless flow of postures (classes might be called *vinyasa* flow, dynamic, or power yoga). If you prefer a more esoteric approach that includes chanting and a focus on breathing, meditation, and energy-raising techniques, look out for Sivananda or Kundalini yoga. If you have an ongoing health problem, try therapeutic Iyengar yoga or Viniyoga, which tailors sequences of poses to suit your particular healing needs. If you are pregnant or postpartum, find a class especially geared for you. What's important is that you find the teacher inspiring and approachable. In the end this matters more than the type of yoga you follow.

A teacher offers hands-on adjustments while you hold a pose, which help you to relax effortlessly into the posture and to let go of held-in tension.

>> **advice** for beginners

Once you are on your mat, following the sequences set out in this book, you'll find the 15 minutes fly by as you focus on getting to know your body and mind better. What is more tricky is maintaining the enthusiasm and motivation to roll out the mat in the first place. These tips may help.

The most important advice a teacher can offer beginners to yoga is to make the time to roll out their mats. Practicing in the same place and at the same time can help maintain motivation. Decide on a time and write it into your daybook, thinking of it as an appointment you cannot miss. Indeed, this may be one of the most important appointments you make during a day since it allows you to devote time to looking after yourself. This not only makes you feel great, it sets you up for success in every other part of your day, whether that includes achieving work tasks or mixing with other people.

Setting practice times

Early morning is traditionally considered the best time of day to practice yoga. Try setting your alarm 30 minutes earlier than usual. Take a shower and then practice in the quiet period before the rest of your household awakes. It is interesting to note how this period of reflection first thing can make your home life feel less stressed.

Late afternoon or early evening make good alternative practice times, especially if you need an energy boost or would like to wind down after a hectic day. Wash before you begin and make sure your stomach is empty: let two hours pass after a meal before you practice.

Planning the session

At the start of any yoga session, spend a few minutes sitting, or lying on your back with your knees bent and feet flat on the floor. Close your

>> **before** you begin

- **Remove your watch**, glasses, and any jewelery that might get in the way of your practice. If you have long hair, tie it back.

- **Gather together your props**, which may include a belt and yoga blocks, a chair or bolsters, plus a blanket to keep you warm in the final relaxation pose.

- **Turn off your phone**, and any other sensory distractions, such as the radio or music.

- **Close the door** and make sure those who share your home know not to disturb you.

eyes and look inside yourself, watching your breath flow in and out completely naturally. Then carefully follow the warm-up exercises before beginning the postures. Allow at least five minutes after finishing the routine to lie in the final relaxation pose that ends all yoga sessions.

Take it slowly

Yoga is all about getting to know your capabilities and limitations—but you have the rest of your life to complete this study. Do not feel pressured to push it too far or too fast in the early weeks and months, and do let go of any thoughts of perfection. Yoga is not competitive.

Follow your breath

Tune into your breath not only at the beginning of each session, but in every posture to see what it tells you about your practice. If your breathing becomes ragged or uneven at any time take it as a sign to ease off a little. When you arrive in a pose, explore whether breathing out any tension makes you feel more comfortable, and whether the in-breath allows you to expand and reach a little farther. With time, breath-awareness will become second nature.

Listen to your body

Honor the messages your body sends. If your knees or lower back hurt, for example, take it as an instruction to refer to the easier version of the posture. Acknowledge your limitations, taking things slowly and not progressing to the stronger stretches in the sequences until fully ready—but do not accept your current limitations as your fate. Yoga encourages us to explore the boundaries of what we can do, and to challenge ourselves, but without pursuing perfection, which may lead to physical injury and to unhelpful emotions such as anger or pride. The key to a fulfilling yoga practice is to let expectations go, but to keep pushing into your "edges." Try to incorporate some yoga poses into your everyday life, for example, practice leg raises while you are on the phone or sit on the floor with your back straight while you are reading or watching television, instead of slouching on the sofa, and you will soon notice a real difference.

Incorporate yoga into your daily activities. Sitting on the floor with your legs stretched out in front of you and a straight back will help improve your posture and aid you in your yoga practice.

>> **practicing** safely

Yoga is about knowing yourself. It is important not to push your body beyond its limits. If some of the postures are difficult to start with, feel pleased that you have a challenge ahead of you. For more difficult poses, there are easier options throughout the book for you to refer to.

If you are not used to doing exercise, it is important that you learn the difference between sweet pain—a good, stretchy feeling in the muscles—and sour, or negative, pain—a sharp or nagging pain. This can take time to understand; go slowly. To begin with, you may feel some stiffness for a day or two afterward, but this will soon pass. Do not force your body into positions that it cannot perform. If you find that a pose creates negative pain or tension in a part of your body, ease off. Always veer to the safe side and modify the pose, referring to the easier option, or use equipment (shown on pp. 314–315) to help you in positions that cause you difficulty.

Always practice yoga on an empty stomach. Allow two to three hours to elapse after a meal before starting yoga.

If you have a specific injury, are pregnant, or have any other health concerns, consult a doctor before using this book. If you feel dizzy, experience chest pain or heart irregularity, or become short of breath while practicing yoga, stop immediately.

Use your environment to help you. Use a shelf for support for a modified standing bend instead of Downward Dog (see p. 321) and a wall or door to lean your legs up against at the end of a tiring day.

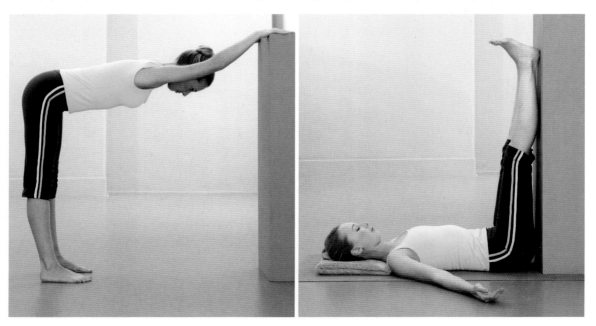

>> **before** you begin

- **Consult** a doctor before practicing yoga if you have an injury, any health concerns, or you are pregnant.

- **Practice** on an empty stomach. Allow three hours to pass after a large meal, two hours after a light meal, and one hour after a snack.

- **Do not overreach** yourself. Take it slowly at first and stop if you are experiencing any negative pain or tension.

- **Refer to the easier options** where relevant and use props to help you in difficult poses.

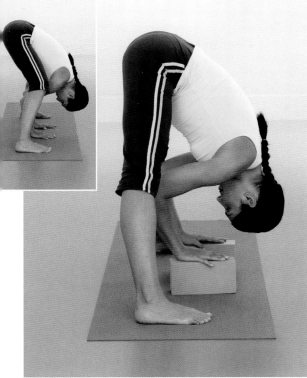

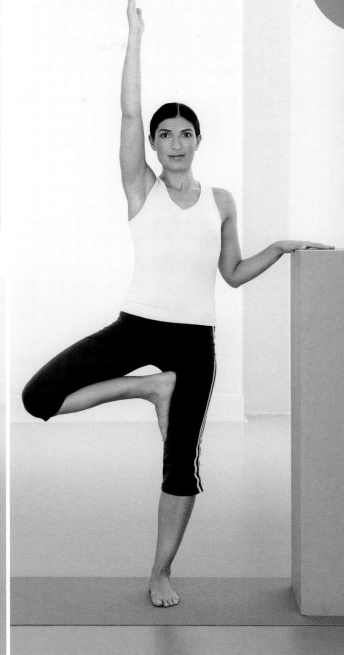

If you find it difficult to reach the floor in a standing forward bend, bend your knees (see inset) or place a block under your hands.

Balancing can be hard at first for beginners or if you are feeling particularly tired. Use a wall to lean against or a surface to hold on to.

>> **clothing** and equipment

There is no need to spend vast amounts of money on specific equipment or clothes. Invest in a yoga mat, but just wear comfortable clothing, and if you need props to help you with the more difficult poses, use household items that have the same effect as the yoga equipment available to buy.

When you are new to yoga, you may find that you need all the help you can get to discipline yourself. It helps if you find a little spot in your home that you can practice in regularly and where you will not be disturbed. Tell the people you share your home with that you want at least 15 minutes of private time. Make sure that the phone is silenced and that you are away from your computer and daily chores. If you use the same place each time for your practice, you may find that it develops a special energy that you associate with your practice. You may feel you want to light a candle, place a bowl of flowers there, or a picture of someone who inspires you.

Practice in a quiet, clean, warm environment. A wooden floor is ideal, or one that allows you to practice without a mat. However, if the surface of the floor is slippery, you must use a yoga mat. As a beginner, you may want to be close to a wall when practicing, to help support you when balancing.

Clothing

Before starting, change into comfortable clothes that do not restrict you in any way. You may also feel you want to wash before you practice. The clothing you wear must be comfortable and flexible, with elastic waist bands. Fabrics that are made from natural fibers work well, since they help the body to breathe. Wear shorts, leggings, cropped pants, or pants that you can roll up, which allow you to see if your legs and feet are correctly aligned. Bare feet are essential so that you are able to stretch out and invigorate your feet.

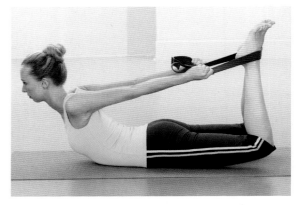

Wrapping a belt around your feet can help you hold a pose that you otherwise may not be able to (see Full Bow, p. 357).

Equipment

If your floor is slippery you will need to buy a yoga mat, but for the other equipment, use general household items that have the same effect. As you become more experienced, you may find that you want to buy equipment specially designed for yoga.

● **Using a belt** helps to deepen a pose without applying force and to hold a pose in correct alignment. You may also need to use one for poses where you are unable to reach your hands together (see Cow Face Pose, p. 349) or to help bring your legs off the floor (see Full Bow, p. 357). You can use a bathrobe belt at first.

mat

● **Blocks** are useful if your hands cannot quite reach the floor, or if you need more height under your sitting bones. Sitting on them also helps keep you straight. Different-sized blocks are available to buy, but you can use telephone books or other books instead. Cover them or tape them up so that they are firmer.

● **Placing a bolster** underneath you when lying flat helps open up your chest. You can also use it to sit on or place it under your knees to relax your back in the final relaxation (see p. 359).

● **Lightweight blankets or towels** are useful to have on hand. These can be folded or rolled up neatly to support you and make you more comfortable when sitting or lying. You can also use them to cover you to keep you warm during relaxation. Place an eye pad over your eyes during the final relaxation.

● **Place a chair or stool** near to you when you are practicing. If you feel particularly stiff and it is difficult for you to take your hands to the floor, use

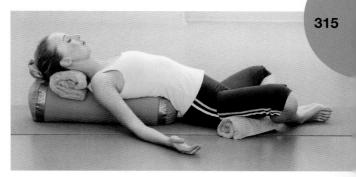

Use a bolster and towels to make you more comfortable. Lying on a bolster also helps open your chest, helping you breathe.

a chair to put your hands on to help you bend over. Use a chair or stool for resting your calves during the final relaxation and also for support when it is hard to balance in the standing poses.

Classic yoga equipment is available from specific yoga stores and online. At first, use household items to help you feel more comfortable and relaxed and to modify the more difficult poses.

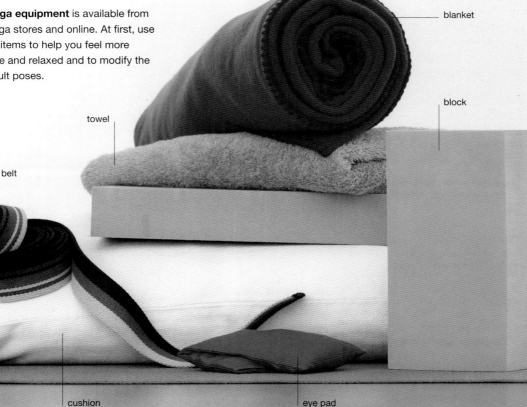

blanket

towel

block

belt

cushion

eye pad

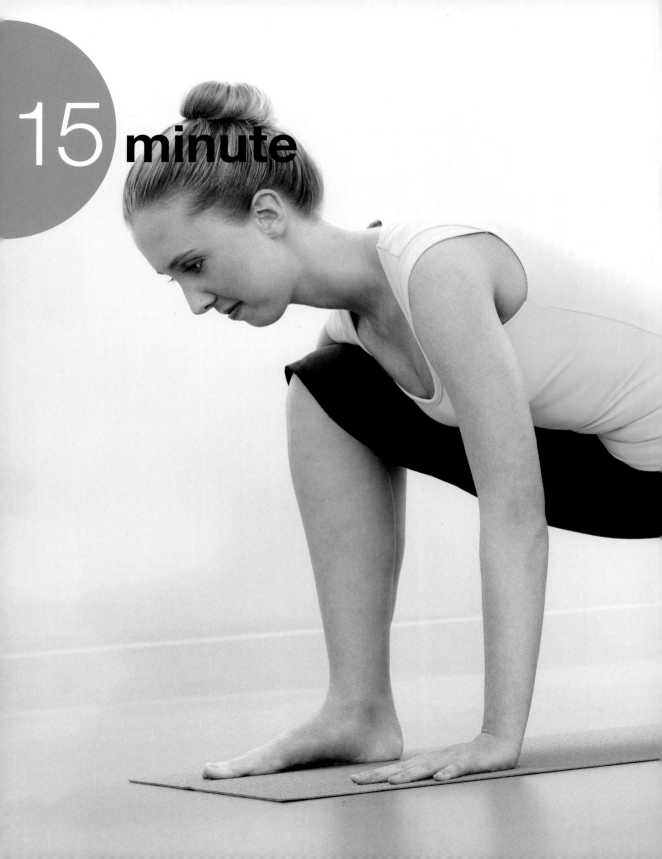

15 minute

rise and shine >>

Start the morning
with a series of gentle,
flowing movements
Prepare yourself for
the day ahead

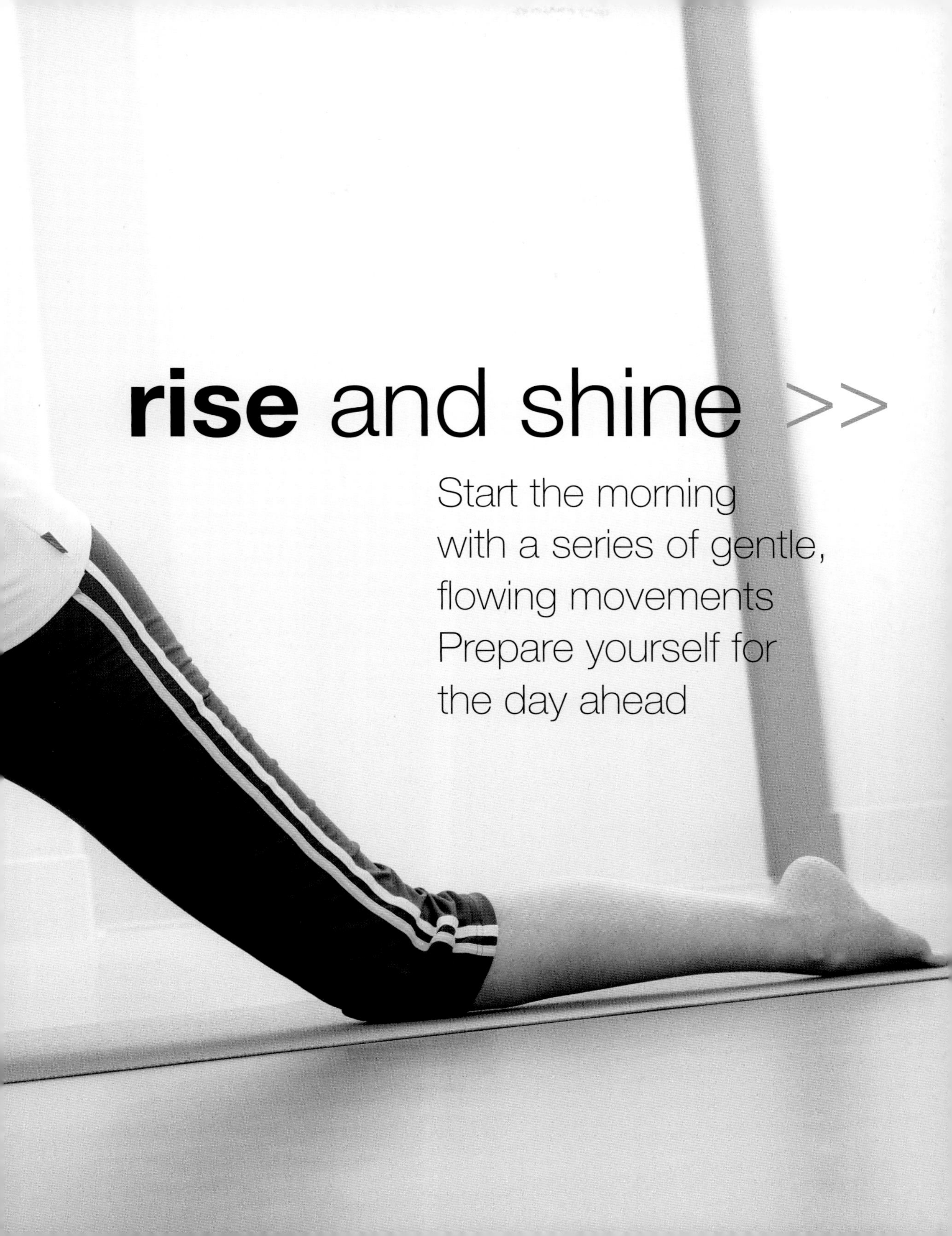

>> listening to your breath

1 Lie flat on your back with your knees bent and your arms out at 45 degrees to your body. Keep the back of your neck long. Close your eyes and listen to your natural breath coming and going. To bring more awareness into your lungs, breathe in steadily for 3 counts and out for 4, repeating several times.

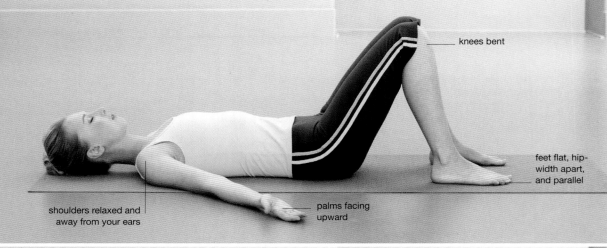

knees bent

feet flat, hip-width apart, and parallel

palms facing upward

shoulders relaxed and away from your ears

2 Inhale and bend your knees toward your chest, with your hands resting on your knees. Keep the back of your neck long.

knees bent towards your body

keep the neck long

3 Exhale and stretch your right leg out along the floor, keeping your leg straight and strong. Flex your foot and keep it about 1 in (2.5 cm) off the floor. Inhale and bend both knees toward your chest. Exhale and repeat with your left leg. Repeat for both legs once more, returning both knees back toward your body (see step 2, opposite).

stretch along the inside of your leg to the inner heel

foot flexed and 1 in (2.5 cm) off the floor

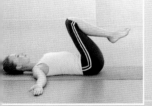

4 Keep your knees bent toward your chest and stretch your arms out to your sides. Exhale and take both knees down toward your right elbow. At the same time, turn your head and abdomen toward the left. Inhale and come back to the center (see inset). Exhale and repeat on your left side, as you turn your head and navel toward the right. Repeat on both sides, returning to the center each time.

head and abdomen turned away from your knees

arms out to the side at shoulder-height

palms facing upward

knee and foot on the floor, if they will go

>> rock and roll/circling

5 Start to awaken the spine. With your knees still hugged toward your body, but holding the back of your knees, gently rock backward and forward on your spine. Inhale as you roll back. Exhale as you roll forward. Repeat several times. If your back feels too stiff, just roll gently from side to side instead.

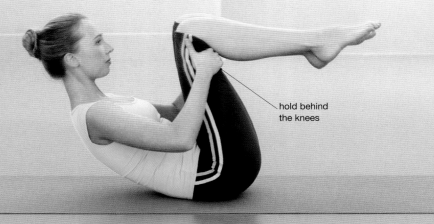

hold behind
the knees

6 Turn to the side to come onto all-fours, facing the front of the mat. Your hands shoulder-width apart, facing forward, and your knees are hip-width apart with the tops of your feet flat on the floor. Circle your hips 3 times to the left, taking one full breath for each circle. Feel like you are drawing a circle with your navel out to your hips. Repeat to the right. Feel your lower back relaxing.

tops of the feet
on the floor

hands shoulder-width
apart and facing
forward

7 Inhale and look ahead. Keep your shoulders away from your ears and your tailbone back (see inset). Exhale, rounding your back and looking to your navel, as you stretch your buttocks back and down toward your heels, with your head resting on the floor for Child's Pose. Your hands are on the floor in front of you. At first, your head may not touch the floor and your buttocks may not reach your heels. If your knees feel very stiff, place a blanket behind the knees. If your ankles hurt, place a rolled towel under them.

buttocks
stretching down
toward the heels

point the
fingers forward

easier option

push the
sitbones up

8 Inhale and come up onto all-fours again, placing your feet flat on the floor. Look ahead. Keep your shoulders away from your ears and draw your navel back to the spine. Exhale and tuck your toes under, as you come up into Downward Dog. Push away and down with your heels and up with your buttocks, lengthening your spine. Bend your knees if your hamstrings feel too tight (see inset). Repeat steps 7–8 once more.

neck relaxed

push the
heels away
and down

straight arms

>> forward bend/extended mountain

9 Gently walk your feet and hands toward each other until you are in a Standing Forward Bend. Your feet are parallel and hip-width apart. If your back feels stiff, keep your legs bent (see inset). Inhale, bending your knees more. Exhale, lifting your kneecaps and sucking the front of your thighs up and back. Feel your feet growing roots down into the floor, relaxed, but grounding down. Breathe freely.

easier option

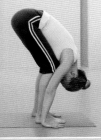

10 Inhale and sweep your arms out to the side and up over your head as you come up to standing for Extended Mountain pose. By the time your arms are over your head, your legs are straight. Stretch all along the outside of your body to your finger tips.

arms reaching up

feet parallel and hip-width apart

feet pushing down

11 Exhale, bringing your arms out and down by your side. Step your feet together at the front of the mat and stand in Mountain pose. Feel a plumb line through the center of your body. Get ready for 2 rounds of Sun Salutation.

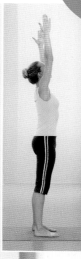

12 Exhale and bring your hands into Prayer Position in front of your chest. Inhale and sweep your arms out and up over your head (see inset). Look up.

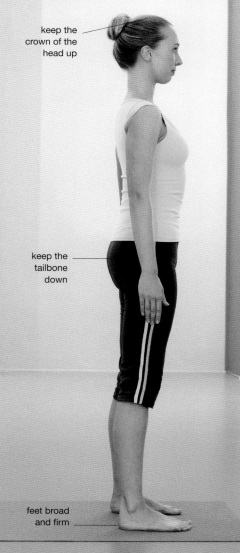

keep the crown of the head up

keep the tailbone down

feet broad and firm

hands in Prayer Position

>> **forward bend/lunge**

13 Exhale and swing your arms out and down as you bend forward into Standing Forward Bend. Place your hands on the floor by the side of your feet, but allow your knees to bend if necessary. Keep your head relaxed.

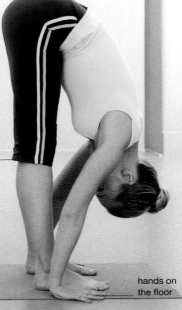

bend the knees if need be

hands on the floor

14 Inhale and bring your right leg back and your knee to the floor. Place your hands on the floor on either side of your front foot for a Lunge.

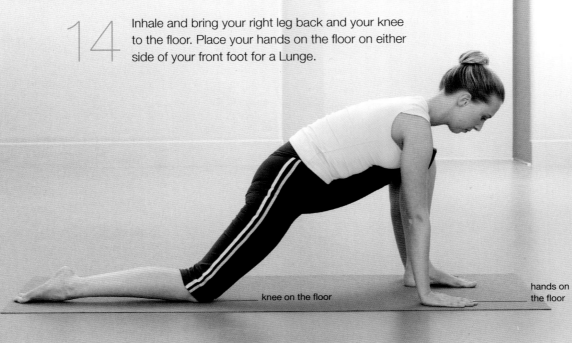

knee on the floor

hands on the floor

>> downward dog/plank

15 Exhale and come back into Downward Dog (see inset). Bend your knees, if need be. Inhale forward into a Plank. Keep your body and arms straight. Push your heels away and the crown of your head forward.

push the crown of the head forward

push the heels away

16 Exhale and bring your knees, chest, and chin down to the floor. Keep your elbows hugged into your sides and your hips high. If this is too hard, bring your feet farther back on the mat.

hips high

elbows close to the body

>> cobra/downward dog

17 Inhale into the Cobra. Keep your elbows hugged into your sides and bring the tops of your feet and legs down onto the floor. Lengthen all along your legs to the inner heel. Push down with your pubic bone and lift your navel to your chest. Keep your shoulders down, away from your ears. Lift upward with the top of your chest. Look ahead. If this is difficult, place your elbows and forearms on the floor in front of you for the Sphinx (see inset).

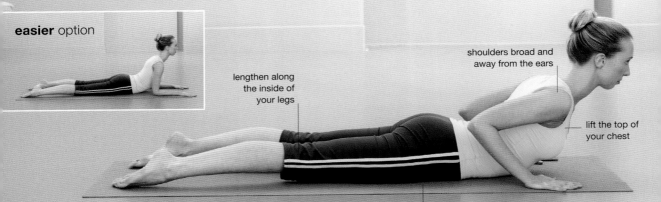

easier option

lengthen along the inside of your legs

shoulders broad and away from the ears

lift the top of your chest

push down with your pubic bone

18 Exhale and tuck your toes under and push up into the Downward Dog. Take a couple of breaths here. Inhale and bring your right foot forward, in between your hands, as you bring your left knee to the floor (see inset). Look ahead. If this is difficult, use your hand to bring the foot forward (see easier option).

push up as high as possible

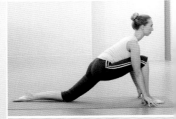

easier option

push the mat back with the balls of the feet

push the mat forward with the hands

19 Exhale and bring your back foot forward to join your front foot. Place your hands on the floor on either side of your feet for a Standing Forward Bend, keeping your knees bent if necessary. Keep your heels firm on the floor, but bring your weight farther forward, so that you can feel your front thigh muscles lifting, the backs of your knees opening, and your calves stretching down to your heels.

20 Sweep your arms out to the side and up over your head as you come back up to standing. Look up. Exhale and bring your hands down the center line to the chest into Prayer Position (see inset). Look ahead. Repeat steps 12–20 on your left side to complete one full round of the Sun Salutation, and then repeat another full round. Bring your hands down by the side of your body for Mountain Pose. Listen to your breath coming and going. Step back to the middle of the mat.

heels firm on the floor

>> child's pose/lion

21 Kneel down to Child's Pose. Allow your big toes to touch, but keep your heels apart. Rest your forehead on the floor and let your sitting bones sink down to your heels. Bring your arms by your feet, palms facing upward. Breathe naturally. As you inhale, you may feel your breath moving in your lower back. Exhale and relax.

toes touching and heels apart

forehead rests on the floor

22 Roll up, vertebra by vertebra, with your head coming up last, until you are sitting up straight for the Lion. Place your hands on your knees. If it is uncomfortable to kneel, place a cushion behind your knees and a rolled towel under your ankles. Inhale. Open your mouth wide and stretch your tongue out; look in between your eyebrows and exhale through your mouth with a roar (a "ha" sound). Inhale and close your eyes and mouth. Repeat twice more.

straight arms

23 Move your hands farther back up your thighs with your palms facing upward. Close your eyes. Breathe in as if you are smelling a beautiful flower. Exhale and let go. Sit quietly, focusing on your breath coming and going.

palms facing upward

24 Lie on your back with your knees bent and your feet flat on the floor (hip-width apart and parallel). Lift your head and look down your center line to see that you are straight. Place your head on the floor and your arms away from your body. Lengthen one leg out along the floor and then the other, ready for the final relaxation. Stay here for 2–5 minutes. Place a folded blanket under your head, a cushion under your knees and an eye pad on your eyes, if you wish, to make you more comfortable.

shoulders relaxed and away from the ears

palms facing upward

rise and shine at a glance

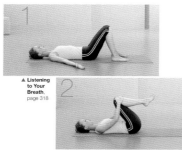

▲ Listening to Your Breath, page 318

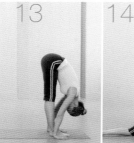

▲ Listening to Your Breath, page 318

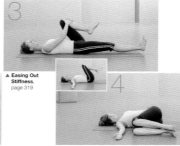

▲ Easing Out Stiffness, page 319

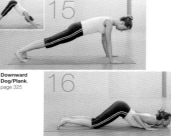

▲ Easing Out Stiffness, page 319

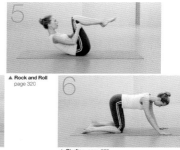

▲ Rock and Roll, page 320

▲ Circling, page 320

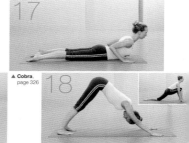

▲ Standing Forward Bend, page 324

▲ Lunge, page 324

▲ Downward Dog/Plank, page 325

▲ Knees, Chest, and Chin to Floor, page 325

▲ Cobra, page 326

▲ Downward Dog/Lunge, page 326

strengthening at a glance

▲ Quietening the Mind, page 334

▲ Shining Skull (Kapalabhati), page 334

▲ Diagonal Stretch, page 335

▲ Plank, page 335

▲ Bent Leg Dog, page 336

▲ Standing Forward Bend, page 336

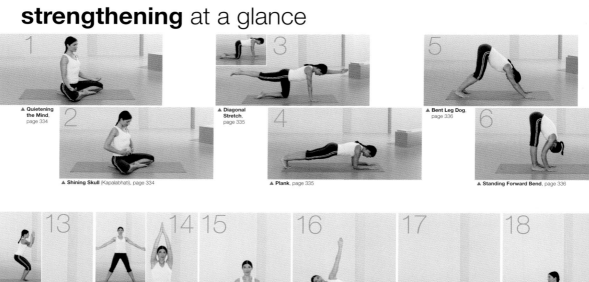

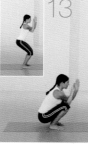

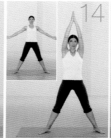

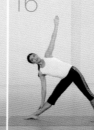

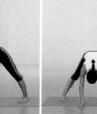

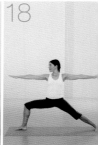

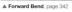

▲ Squat, page 340

▲ Preparation for Horse, page 340

▲ Horse, page 341

▲ Triangle, page 341

▲ Forward Bend, page 342

▲ Warrior 2, page 342

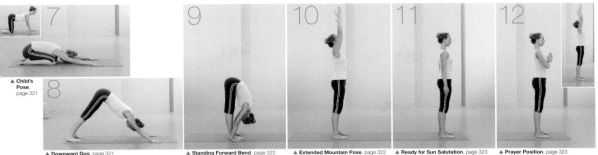

▲ Child's Pose, page 321

▲ Downward Dog, page 321

▲ Standing Forward Bend, page 322

▲ Extended Mountain Pose, page 322

▲ Ready for Sun Salutation, page 323

▲ Prayer Position, page 323

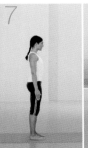
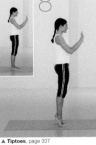
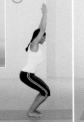
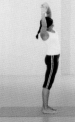
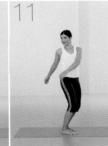

▲ Standing Forward Bend, page 327

▲ Sun Salutation, page 327 Repeat 12–20

▲ Child's Pose, page 328

▲ Lion, page 328

▲ Final Relaxation, page 329

▲ Final Relaxation, page 329

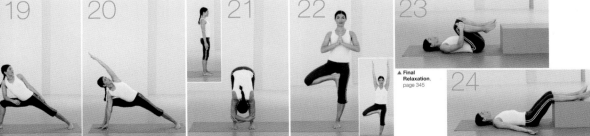

▲ Mountain Pose, page 337

▲ Tiptoes, page 337

▲ Chair Pose, page 338

▲ Standing Lateral Stretch, page 338

▲ Standing Rhythmic Twist, page 339

▲ Eagle Arms, page 339

▲ Side Angle Stretch, page 343

▲ Side Angle Stretch, page 343

▲ Standing Forward Bend, page 344

▲ Tree Pose, page 344

▲ Final Relaxation, page 345

▲ Final Relaxation, page 345

15 minute

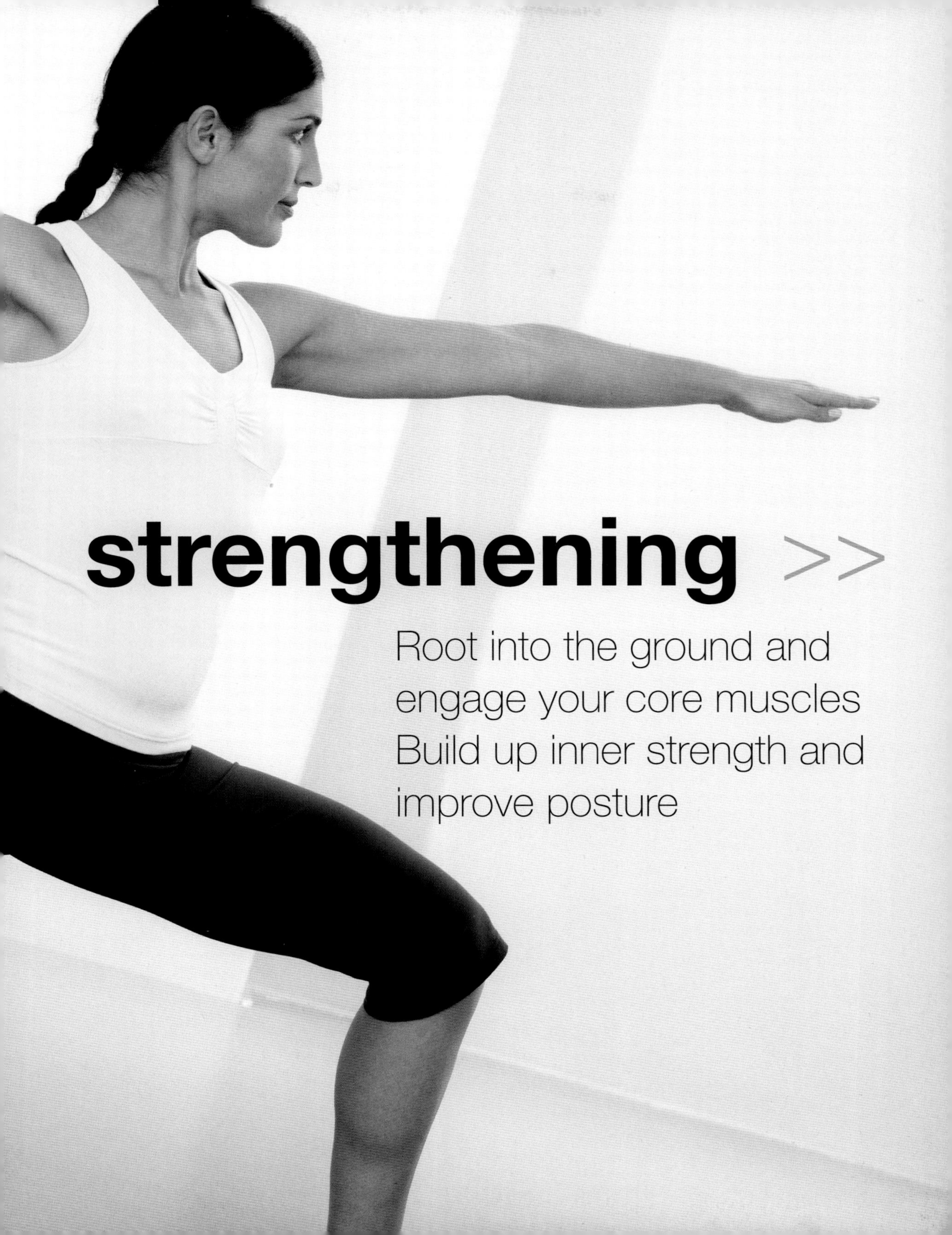

strengthening >>

Root into the ground and
engage your core muscles
Build up inner strength and
improve posture

>> quieting the mind/shining skull

1 Sit cross-legged on a block or cushion with your back straight and your hands resting on your knees or thighs. If it is difficult to sit straight, make your base higher. If your knees don't touch the floor, put cushions under your thighs. Watch your breath and allow your mind to quiet.

shoulders relaxed

elbows slightly bent

palms facing upward

sit on a block or cushion

2 Remain cross-legged for Shining Skull (Kapalabhati), an exercise to cleanse the lungs and mind. Concentrate on a strong exhalation as you pull your abdomen in and then immediately allow it to relax so that the inhalation (see inset) is spontaneous and relaxed. Repeat 10 pumps quickly. Return to natural inhalation and exhalation for a few breaths before each round. Repeat twice.

contract abdominal muscles quickly on exhalation

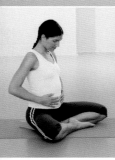

3 Come onto all fours (see inset) for a Diagonal Stretch. Exhale and stretch your left arm forward and your right leg back. Keep your shoulders away from your ears and your leg straight and strong. Draw your abdomen back to the spine to support your lower back. Inhale and come back to the center. Repeat on your other side and repeat again on both sides.

abdomen is drawing back to the spine

hands are in line with the shoulders

knees are in line with hips

4 For a Plank, bring your elbows down to the floor, in line with your shoulders. Place your forearms straight out in front of you on the floor. Exhale and lift your knees off the floor, pushing your heels back and away. Your body should be straight. Draw your abdomen back to the spine. Keep your shoulders away from your ears, your neck long and the crown of your head forward. Breathe naturally.

push the heels back and away

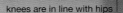

navel is pulling back to the spine

forearms are shoulder-width apart

>> bent leg dog/forward bend

push the sitbones up

5 Come back onto all-fours, tucking your toes under. Exhale, lifting your knees off the floor and straightening your legs into Downward Dog. Push your sitbones up, relax your head, and keep your arms straight. If your hamstrings feel very tight initially, bend your legs, feeling your spine lengthening. On every exhalation, pull the front of your thighs up to help straighten your legs.

push the mat forward with the hands

push the mat back with the balls of the feet

6 Walk your hands and feet toward each other into a Standing Forward Bend. If your hamstrings feel tight, bend your knees a little (see inset). Over time, as your sitbones shoot up and your feet grow roots down, your legs will gently straighten. If your back hurts at all, bend your knees more or rest your hands on a chair or shelf in a Half Forward Bend (see p. 312).

easier option

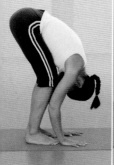

7 Roll up, vertebra by vertebra, until you are in Mountain Pose. Stand with your feet hip-width apart, growing roots down. Draw your abdomen back to the spine. Breathe through your nose, feeling your breath softly caressing the back of your throat.

8 For the Tiptoes exercise, bring your hands in front of you at shoulder height with your palms facing forward and your elbows by your side. Inhale and come up onto the balls of your feet. Exhale and come down. Repeat 4 times.

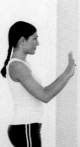

keep the crown of the head up

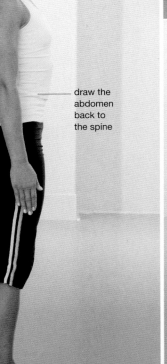

draw the abdomen back to the spine

keep the tailbone down

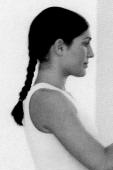

place the hands against a wall if balancing is difficult

bring the heels up high as you come up onto the tiptoes

9 Inhale and move your arms forward and up over your head as you come onto your tiptoes. Stretch up to your fingertips (see inset). Exhale, bringing your heels down, and bend your knees into the Chair Pose. Inhale, straightening your legs. Exhale, and bring your arms out and down by your side.

arms stay above the head for Chair Pose

10 Interlace your fingers for a Standing Lateral Stretch. Turn your hands out and push your palms away from you. Inhale, lifting your arms up over your head. Exhale, stretching to the right, with a firm weight on your left foot. Inhale back to the center. Repeat to the left. Change the interlace of your fingers. Repeat once more on both sides.

root down with the opposite foot

11 Bring your arms out and down, ready for Standing Rhythmic Twist. With your knees slightly bent and your arms hanging loosely by your side, swing your upper body from left to right. Your arms are relaxed and gently swinging from side to side with your hands tapping your body. Breathe naturally as you rhythmically swing.

12 For Eagle Arms, lift your arms out to the side and wrap your right arm over your left. Place the fingers of your left hand into your right palm, and bring your thumbs in front of your nose. Push forward with your left hand and pull back with your right.

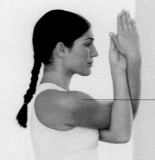

shoulders away from the ears

arms relaxed and gently swinging

>> squat/preparation for horse

13 Exhale down into a Squat. Feel the weight on the outside of your feet. If it is difficult to squat, just come down as far as you are able, without lifting your heels (see inset). Inhale and come back up. Exhale and release your arms out to the side. Switch hands and repeat. Inhale and come up, releasing your arms out and down by your side.

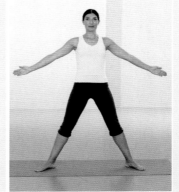

14 Step around to the middle of the mat. Move your feet wide apart and turn them out to 45 degrees (see inset). Inhale and bring your arms out and up over your head, palms touching.

knees over the feet

tailbone down

feet just wider than hip-width apart

feet wide and turned out at 45 degrees

15 Exhale into the Horse, bending your knees so that they are in line with your feet and bringing your hands down through your center line into Prayer Position. Inhale and push your feet into the floor to straighten your legs. Bring your arms over your head as you come up. Touch your palms together above your head. Repeat once more.

16 Inhale and straighten your legs. Stretch your arms out straight at shoulder height. Turn your right foot out and your left foot in for Triangle pose. Exhale out to the right, bringing your right hand to rest on your right shin, and your left arm up, straight. Inhale and look down at your front big toe. Exhale and look ahead. Take a couple of breaths here, come up, and repeat on the left side.

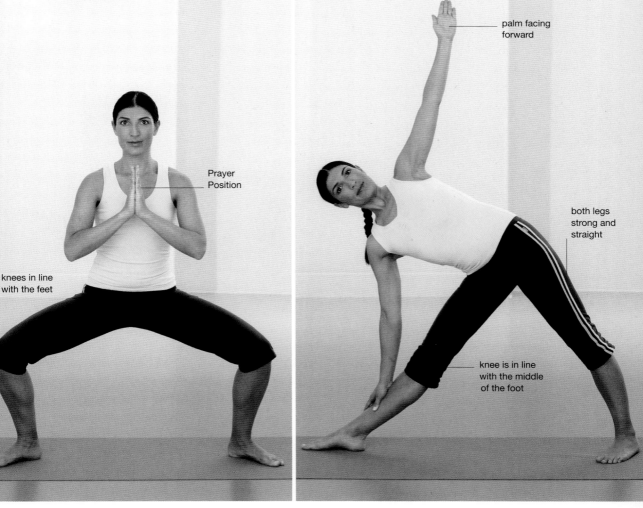

palm facing forward

Prayer Position

both legs strong and straight

knees in line with the feet

knee is in line with the middle of the foot

>> forward bend/warrior 2

17 Inhale and come back up to center. For a Wide Leg Forward Bend, rest your hands on your hips. Inhale and look up. Exhale and hinge at your hips, bringing your hands down to the floor. Bend your knees a little, if need be, or use blocks to rest your hands on (see p. 313, bottom left picture). Walk your feet a little wider apart. Inhale and look ahead. Exhale, let your head go, and bring your hands farther back, in line with your toes (see inset). Inhale and look ahead. Exhale and bring your hands to your hips. Inhale and come up.

feet parallel

hands in line with the shoulders

18 Turn your right foot out and keep your left foot in, ready for Warrior 2. Exhale and bend your right knee directly over your ankle. Rotate both your knees away from each other. Keep strong and straight on your left leg all the way to the outside of your foot. Inhale and stretch your arms out, looking out toward your right index finger. Have a couple of breaths here.

arms out at shoulder height

calf forms a right angle with the thigh

rotate the knee out

19 For a modified Side Angle Stretch, place your right elbow onto your right knee, resting your left hand on the outside of your left thigh. Turn your abdomen and chest up toward the ceiling. Look up at your left shoulder as your right elbow pushes your right knee back and you roll your right buttock under. Feel the stretch through your straight back leg to the outside of your foot. Breathe freely.

leg is straight
and strong to
the outside of
the foot

20 If you want to go further, inhale and stretch your left arm out and up over your head, as you bring your right hand to the floor on the inside of your right foot. Hit your right knee back with your right elbow and roll your right buttock under as you turn your torso upward. Have a couple of breaths here. Inhale and come back up. Repeat steps 18–20 on your left side.

keep a straight line
from the left foot to
the fingertips

>> standing forward bend/tree pose

21 Inhale and come back up, bringing your arms down by your side (see inset). Stand with your feet hip-width apart, in Mountain Pose. With your hands on your hips, hinge forward into a Standing Forward Bend. Hold your elbows and release forward. Take a couple of breaths. Inhale and look ahead. Exhale and place your hands on your hips. Inhale and come up with a flat back to Mountain Pose with your arms by your side.

22 Step your feet together for Tree Pose. Place the sole of your right foot on your inner left thigh. Move your hands into Prayer Position. If you want to go further, inhale and take your arms over your head (see inset). Bring your arms down through the center line to Prayer Position. Release your right foot. Bring your feet together and repeat on the other side. If it is difficult to balance, stand next to a wall.

bend the knees a little, if this is difficult

press the foot into the thigh and the thigh into your foot

23 Take your chair or stool and place it at the end of the mat. Lie down in front of the chair or stool, with your knees bent toward your chest for a Back Release exercise. Hold your knees with your hands. Exhale and hug your knees toward your chest. Inhale and release. Repeat a couple of times.

knees hugged toward the chest

24 For the Final Relaxation, bring your arms down by your side and rest your calves on the chair or stool. Check that you are straight and close your eyes. Place a blanket under your head if it is more comfortable, and an eye pad on your eyes. Stay here for 2–5 minutes.

neck is long

shoulders relaxed, away from the ears

palms facing upward

15 minute

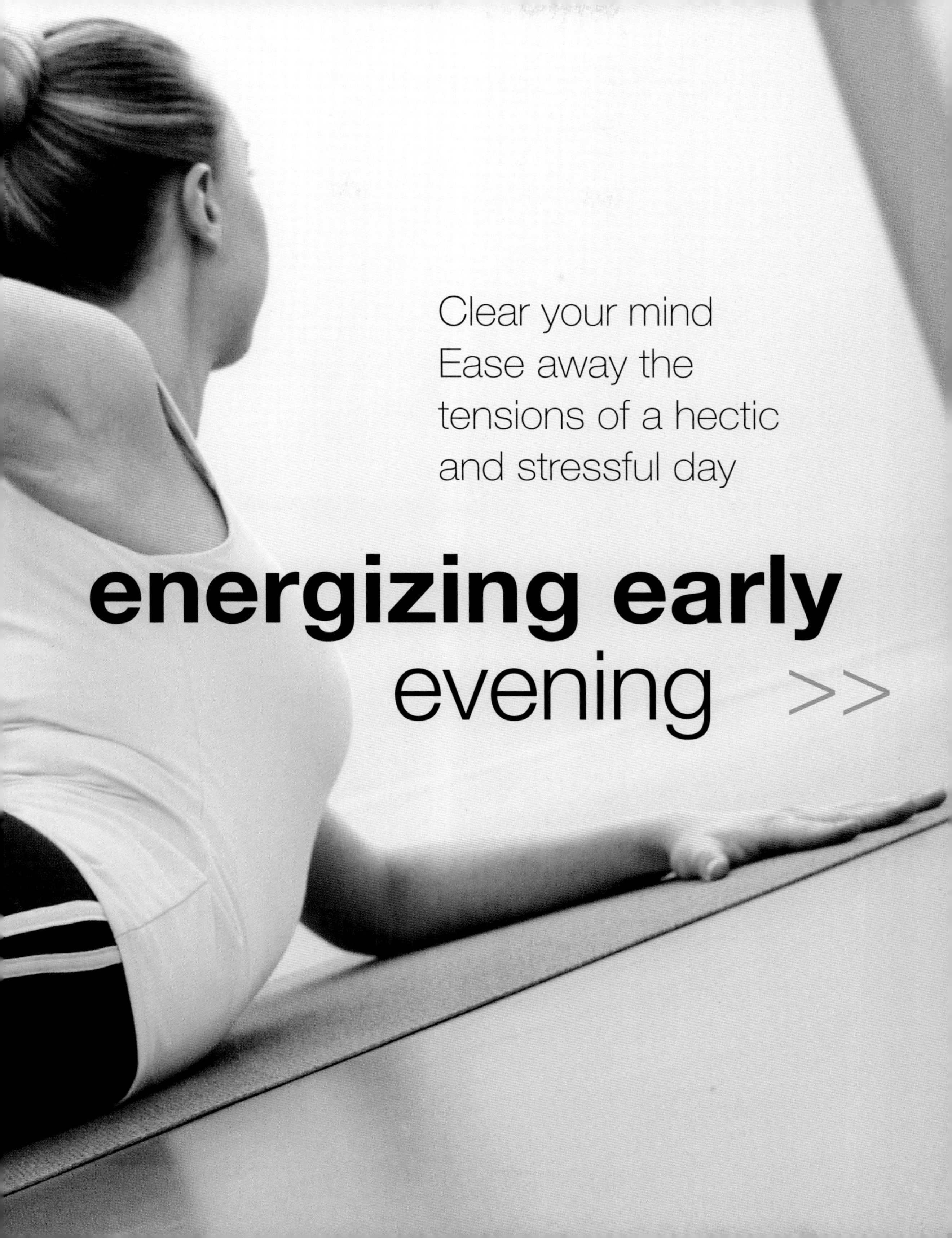

Clear your mind
Ease away the
tensions of a hectic
and stressful day

energizing early
evening >>

1 Sit cross-legged, ready for Alternate Nostril Breathing. Rest your hands on your thighs with your palms facing upward. Bring the tips of your index fingers and thumbs together for Chin Mudra. Close your eyes and watch your natural breath.

eyes closed

index finger and thumb touching

2 On your right hand, bend the index and middle fingers down (see top inset), so that your thumb is free to close your right nostril, and your ring and little fingers are together, ready to close your left nostril. Inhale through both nostrils. Block your right nostril (see bottom inset). Exhale through the left for 4 counts. Inhale through the left for 4 counts. Change, blocking the left nostril. Exhale through the right. Inhale through the right. Change and exhale through the left to complete a full round. Do 2 more rounds.

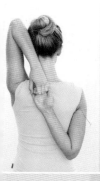

easier option

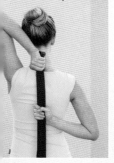

3 Come up to kneeling and bring your arms into Cow Face pose. Take your right hand behind and up your back. Bring your left arm up by your head, bending the elbow so that your forearm comes down your back to clasp the fingers of your right hand (see inset). If this is difficult, use a belt (see easier option). Feel your abdomen drawing back to the spine to support your lower back. Stay for a couple of breaths. Release your arms and repeat on the other side.

4 Stay kneeling, but tuck your toes under and sit on your heels. Exhale and interlace your fingers, stretching your arms out in front of you. Inhale and lift your arms up over your head, keeping them straight. It is common for the toes to hurt a little here, but you should not experience any knee pain. Stay in this pose for just a few seconds at first.

hands reaching up

head is straight

elbows are stretching away from each other

abdomen is drawing back to the spine

sitbones down on the heels

5 Exhale, releasing your hands. With your left hand on your right thigh and your right hand behind you on your left buttock, twist to the right. Inhale, moving back to the center. Change the interlace of your fingers and repeat steps 4 and 5, twisting to the left. If your toes are too painful, put your feet flat again and build up gradually to sitting on your heels.

6 Still kneeling, put your feet flat again. Inhale and move your shoulders forward and up. Exhale, moving them back and down. Repeat twice more. Reverse, moving back and up as you inhale and forward and down as you exhale. Repeat twice more.

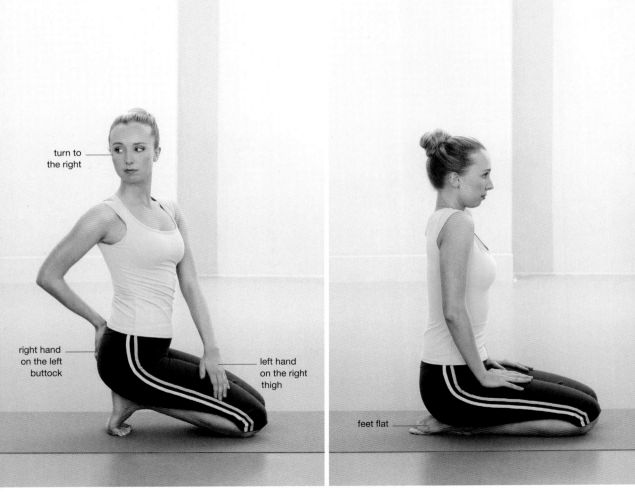

turn to the right

right hand on the left buttock

left hand on the right thigh

feet flat

7 Come up onto all fours with your hands in line with your shoulders and your knees in line with your hips. Keep your neck long and your shoulders broad and away from your ears. Feel your abdomen drawing back to the spine.

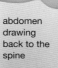

abdomen drawing back to the spine

knees in line with the hips

hands in line with the shoulders

8 Step your right foot forward in between your hands for Lunge. Keep your front shin perpendicular to the floor. If your back knee is hurting on the floor, place a folded towel under it. Sink your hips, stretching your back leg more.

stretch the leg back

fingers touching the floor

>> lunge/downward dog

9 Bring both hands onto your front knee. Exhale, increasing the stretch on your back leg. Feel a strong stretch on your back thigh. Inhale, placing your hands on the floor by your front foot. Exhale and come back onto all fours (see inset). Repeat on the other side. Come back onto all-fours.

shoulders down and broad

feel a strong stretch on your quadricep

10 Inhale, tucking your toes under. Exhale, drawing your abdomen toward your spine and lifting your pelvis to form an inverted "V" with your body in the Downward Dog. Keep your arms and legs straight and turn your armpits to face each other. Push your buttocks up and stretch back and down with your heels, keeping your breath even and smooth.

push the sitting bones up

keep the legs straight, if possible

keep the arms straight

11 Inhale and come back onto your knees. Exhale and lie on your stomach with your forehead on the floor and your arms stretched out in front of you.

12 Exhale, lifting and stretching your right arm and left leg and bringing your head just off the floor. Inhale, bring them back down to the floor. Exhale and repeat on your other side. Repeat again on both sides. Make sure you stretch all along the inside of your leg to the heel. As you stretch your arm forward, keep your shoulders away from your ears.

shoulders away from the ears and broad

>> **rest/locust**

13 Rest. Place your arms by your side with your palms by your hips, facing upward. Turn your head to one side. Lie with your big toes touching and your heels facing out. Close your eyes and focus on even, gentle breathing.

big toes
touching,
heels apart

14 Inhale, bringing your head back to the center. Stretch your hands back toward your toes. Keep your feet and legs firmly on the floor as you exhale, peeling your nose, chin, head and shoulders off the floor in the Locust pose. Breathe evenly. As long as there is no pain in your lower back, lift a little higher. Inhale and relax your body down.

keep the
neck long

feet pushing
down into
the floor

15 If you want to work a little harder, exhale, lifting your straight legs as well as your head and shoulders off the floor. Stretch your arms back toward your feet. Inhale and come down. Repeat (as long as you are not experiencing any back pain).

stretch the arms back
toward the feet

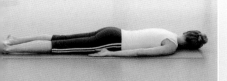

16 Rest, as you did in step 13, but turn your head the other way (see inset). For a Quadriceps Stretch, place your left forearm on the floor in front of you. Lift your head. Bend your right leg and, with your right hand on top of your right foot, stretch your right foot down toward the floor on the outside of your right hip. Breathe evenly.

forearm rests
horizontally in
front of you

pubic bone pushing
into the floor

navel lifting toward
the chest

>> half bow/rest

17 Inhale and move your hand to hold the outside of your right ankle, ready for a Half Bow. Keep both hip bones on the floor. Exhale and lift your right thigh up off the floor. Breathe evenly. Inhale and release down. Repeat steps 16 and 17 on your left side.

lift the thigh up off the floor | keep the hip bones on the floor

18 Make a pillow with your hands in front of you and rest your forehead on your hands. Lie with your big toes touching and your heels apart. Rest, breathing gently.

big toes touching

easier option

19 To do the Full Bow, bend both knees up and hold your ankles firmly with your hands. Exhale and lift your thighs up off the floor. Inhale and, as long as there is no pain in your lower back, lift a little higher as you exhale. Inhale and come down. Use a belt if you find this difficult (see inset).

20 Bring your hands under your shoulders (see inset), exhale, and push back into Child's Pose. Your heels are apart and your big toes are touching. Bring your head to the floor and feel your buttocks stretching down toward your heels. Bring your hands by your feet with your palms facing upward. Breathe in and feel the breath move in your lower back. Exhale and release your buttocks back and down toward your heels. Follow your natural breath.

palms facing
upward

forehead on the floor

>> lord of the fishes twist

21 Inhale, rolling up vertebra by vertebra, with your head coming up last, until you are sitting on your heels. To do the Lord of the Fishes Twist, sit on your left side with your feet out to the right. Place your right foot on the floor, on the outside of your left knee. Rest your left elbow on your right knee. Inhale and feel yourself getting taller. Exhale and turn to the right. Inhale and feel yourself getting taller. Exhale and turn to the right.

right hand on the floor behind you

sitbones push down

easier option

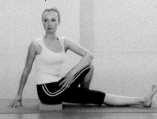

22 Inhale and come back to the center. Repeat on your other side. If you find this twist difficult, place a block underneath you and stretch one leg out in front of you, crossing your other leg over it, bringing the opposite elbow round the top knee (see inset). Inhale and come back to the center. Release your legs out in front of you.

twist as far as possible

fingers touching the floor or a block

foot flat on the floor

23 Lie flat on your back and check that you are straight. Place your right foot behind your left knee. Hold your right thigh with your left hand as you take your right knee toward the floor on the left. Looking out toward the right, let your right arm release to the floor and feel the stretch through your right shoulder and armpit. Inhale and come back to center. Release your legs and repeat on your other side (see inset).

turn the head
to the right

right foot is behind
the left knee

24 Inhale and come back to the center. Lie flat with your knees bent and your feet on the floor (hip-width apart and parallel). Lift your head and look down your center line to see that you are straight. Place your head on the floor and your arms away from your body. Lengthen one leg out along the floor and then the other, ready for the Final Relaxation. Close your eyes and stay here for 2–5 minutes. Place a folded blanket under your head, a cushion under your knees and an eye pad on your eyes, if you wish, to make you more comfortable.

shoulders relaxed and
away from the ears

palms facing upward

energizing early evening at a glance

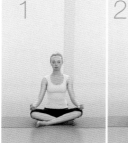

1

▲ Chin Mudra, page 348

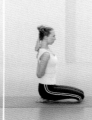

2

▲ Alternate Nostril Breathing, page 348

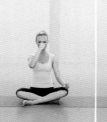

3

▲ Kneeling Pose, page 349

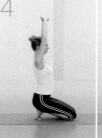

4

▲ Kneeling Pose, page 349

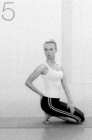

5

▲ Kneeling Pose, page 350

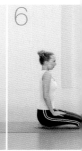

6

▲ Shoulder Rolls, page 350

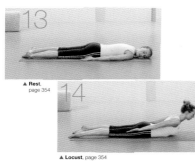

13

▲ Rest, page 354

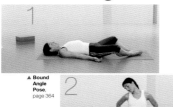

14

▲ Locust, page 354

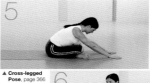

15

▲ Locust/Rest, page 355

16

▲ Quadriceps Stretch, page 355

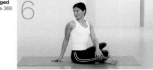

17

▲ Half Bow, page 356

18

▲ Rest, page 356

winding down at a glance

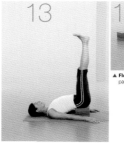

1

▲ Bound Angle Pose, page 364

2

▲ Neck Rolls, page 364

3

▲ Cross-legged Pose, page 365

4

▲ Side-Angle Stretch, page 365

5

▲ Cross-legged Pose, page 366

6

▲ Twist, page 366

13

▲ Bridge, page 370

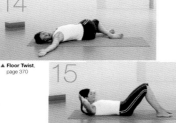

14

▲ Floor Twist, page 370

15

▲ Final Relaxation, page 371

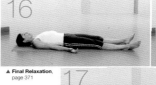

16

▲ Final Relaxation, page 371

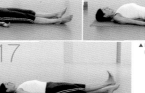

17

▲ Final Relaxation, page 372

18

▲ Final Relaxation, page 372

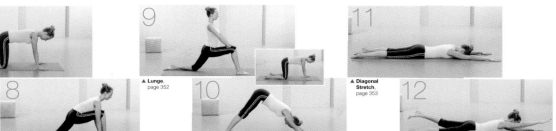

7 ▲ **All Fours**, page 351

8 ▲ **Lunge**, page 351

9 ▲ **Lunge**, page 352

10 ▲ **Downward Dog**, page 352

11 ▲ **Diagonal Stretch**, page 353

12 ▲ **Diagonal Stretch**, page 353

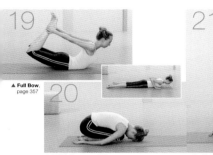

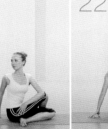

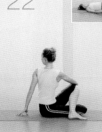

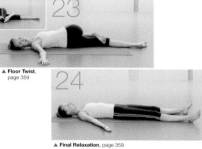

19 ▲ **Full Bow**, page 357

20 ▲ **Child's Pose**, page 357

21 ▲ **Lord of the Fishes Twist**, page 358

22 ▲ **Lord of the Fishes Twist**, page 358

23 ▲ **Floor Twist**, page 359

24 ▲ **Final Relaxation**, page 359

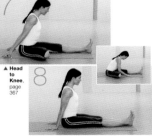

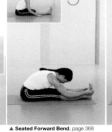

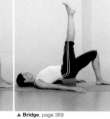

7 ▲ **Head to Knee**, page 367

8 ▲ **Seated Forward Bend**, page 367

9 ▲ **Seated Forward Bend**, page 368

10 ▲ **Hug Knees**, page 368

11 ▲ **Bridge**, page 369

12 ▲ **Bridge**, page 369

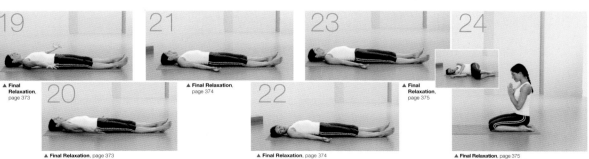

19 ▲ **Final Relaxation**, page 373

20 ▲ **Final Relaxation**, page 373

21 ▲ **Final Relaxation**, page 374

22 ▲ **Final Relaxation**, page 374

23 ▲ **Final Relaxation**, page 375

24 ▲ **Final Relaxation**, page 375

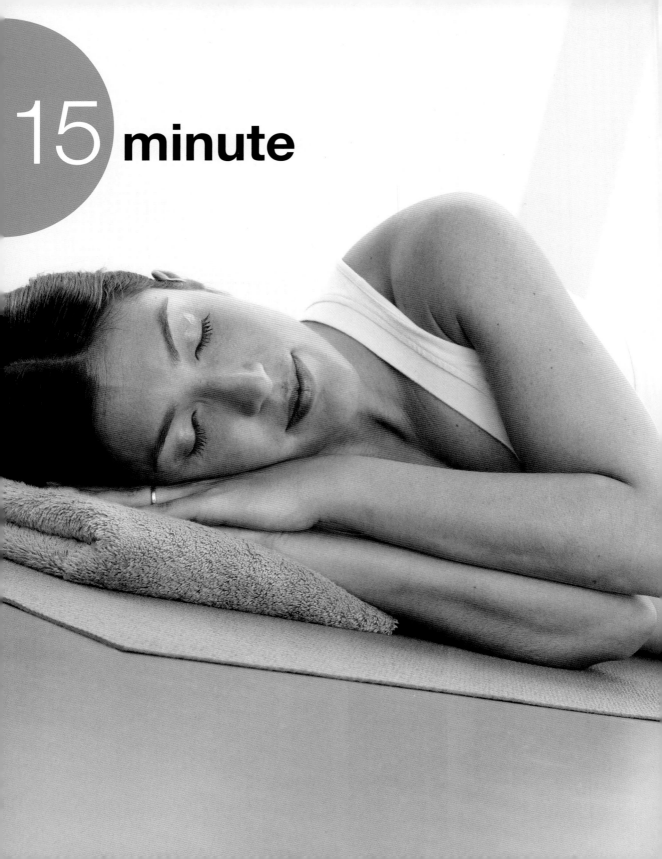

15 minute

winding
down >>

Watch your breath
become slower and
deeper
Prepare for a restful
night's sleep

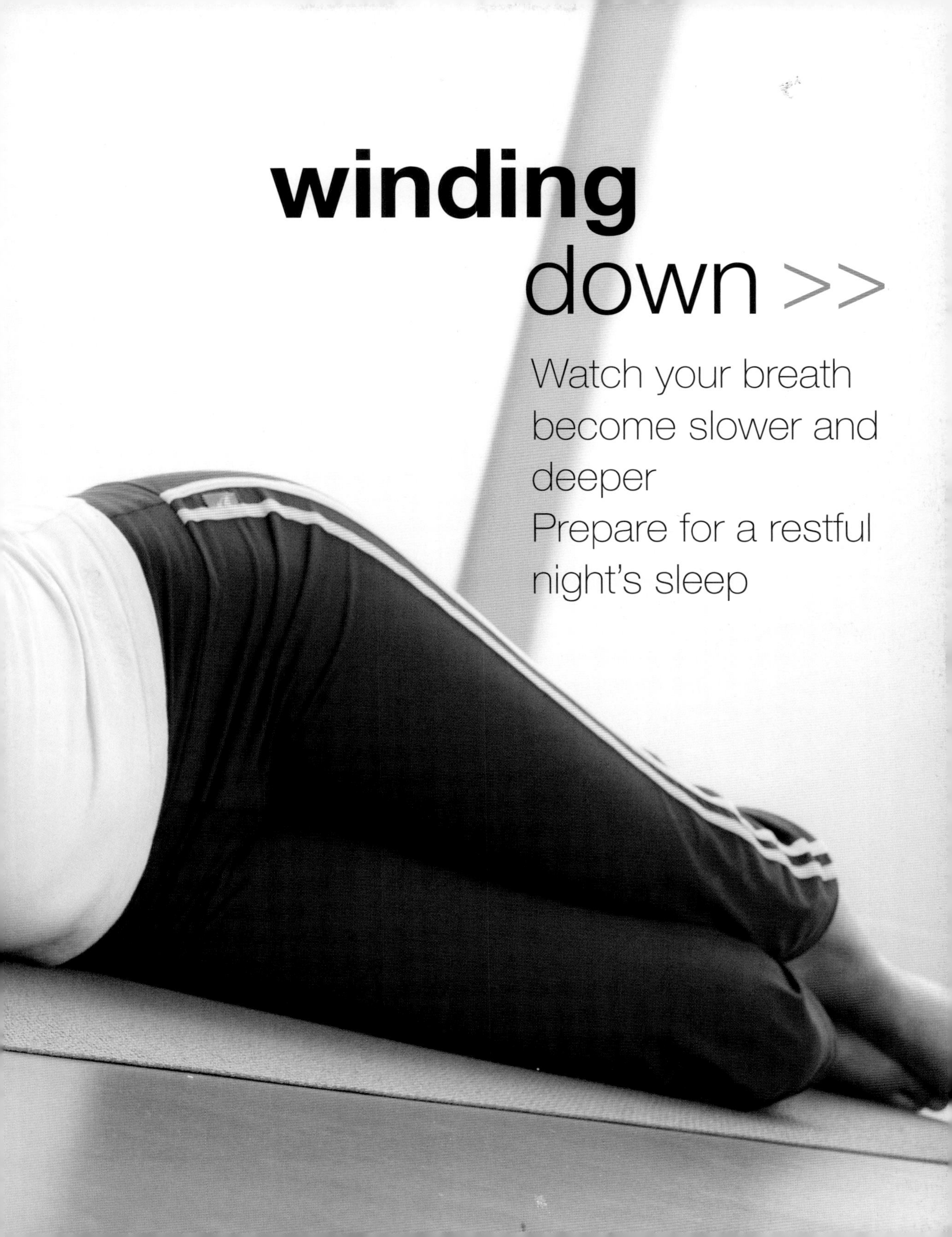

easier option

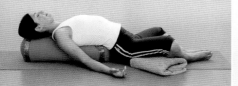

1 Lie flat on your back with the soles of your feet together for Bound Angle Pose. If you like, place blankets and a bolster underneath you to help open your chest (see inset). Close your eyes and follow a breathing circuit: breathe in and wash the brain with the inhalation. Exhale down your spine to your tailbone. Inhale up your spine to in between your eyebrows. Exhale through both your nostrils. Repeat this circuit once more.

soles of the feet together

arms away from the body, palms facing upward

if your neck feels tight, make the circles smaller

2 Roll to the side and come up to sitting on your heels. Place your hands on your waist for Neck Rolls. Imagine you are drawing a circle with the crown of the head. Bring your chin down toward your chest. Inhale as you move your head to the right and back. Exhale as you move to the left and forward (see inset). Repeat and then reverse.

hands on the waist

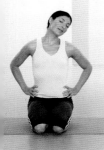

easier option

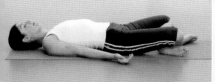

3 Release your legs forward and sit cross-legged. Push down and back with your sitbones and extend your torso over your thighs. Put your hands on the floor in front of you. With each exhalation, stretch forward with your fingers and push down and back with your sitting bones. Breathe naturally. If it is too difficult to come forward, lie on your back with your legs crossed (see inset).

shoulders relaxed and away from the ears

inch forward on each exhalation

4 Inhale and come back up for a Side Angle Stretch. Place your right hand on the floor by your right hip. Keep your elbow bent and shoulder relaxed. Inhale and sweep your left arm up and over your head. Exhale, feeling the stretch on your left side. Inhale and exhale, feeling the stretch. Keep your breathing relaxed. Inhale and come back to the center. Repeat on the other side.

keep the head relaxed

sitbones firm on the floor

>> cross-legged pose/twist

5 Inhale and change the cross of your legs. Relax forward again, as your sitbones push down and back and your fingers inch forward on every exhalation. Let go. On each exhalation, let your torso hinge forward over your thighs to open the hips. If your knees hurt, push back and down with your buttocks and do not come so far forward.

inch forward on every exhalation

root down and back

6 Inhale and come up. Place your left hand on your right thigh and your right hand on the floor behind you, and turn your head and torso to the right. As you inhale, feel yourself getting taller. Exhale, twisting. Inhale and come back to the center. Repeat on the left side.

turn the head and torso to the right

7 Release your legs out in front of you. Bend your right knee and place your foot against the inside of your left thigh. If your knee is not resting on the floor, place a support under the thigh. Keep your left leg straight. Inhale, sit up, and look forward. Place your fingers on the floor behind you. Exhale and come down over your straight leg, bringing your hands to the floor on either side of your leg (see inset). Inhale and come up. Release your right leg out and repeat on the other side.

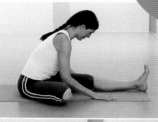

feel even weight through the hands

8 Inhale and come up. Stretch both legs out in front of you. Place your hands on the floor behind you. Sit up. As you push down with your sitbones, feel yourself getting taller. Sit on a support if your back is weak and hold a belt around your feet to help you sit up straight.

>> **seated forward bend/hug knees**

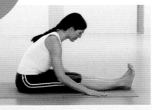

9 Move your hands forward on either side of your legs, as you hinge forward at your hips (see inset). Feel an even weight through both hands. On every exhalation, coming down until, over time, you can clasp both feet.

legs straight

10 Inhale, come up, and lie flat on the floor. With your hands clasped around your knees, hug your knees toward your body. Lift your pelvic floor muscles. As you exhale, lift the pelvic floor. As you inhale, release. Repeat several times.

knees hugged toward the body

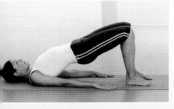

11 Place your feet flat on the floor, hip-width apart. Place your arms on the floor, stretching toward your feet. As you exhale, peel your lower back off the floor, lifting your hips and chest up as your feet grow roots down (see inset). This is the Bridge pose. Place the blocks under your hips. If your back hurts, place fewer blocks beneath you and lengthen your tailbone toward your knees.

feet, knees, and
legs parallel

feet flat

head and shoulders
on the floor

12 Stay as you are, with your hips heavy on the blocks, your chest lifting, and your feet firm on the floor. If there is any pain in your lower back, take a block out. If you want to go further, bend your right knee toward your chest and stretch your right leg straight up. Your left foot remains firm on the floor and your hips are even. Breathe naturally. Inhale and bring your right foot back down to the floor. Repeat with your left leg.

straight leg,
reaching up to
the ceiling

foot flat on the floor
and straight

>> bridge/floor twist

13 If you want to go further, bend both knees toward your chest and stretch both legs straight up. Your hips are heavy on the blocks and your chest is lifting. Return your feet to the floor. Lift your hips off the blocks and take the blocks out, slowly releasing your back down to the floor. Hug your knees toward your chest.

chest lifting

hips heavy on the blocks

14 Stretch your legs out in front of you for a Floor Twist. Wrap your right leg over your left leg and take both legs down to the floor on your left, holding your right thigh with your left hand. Release your right arm out to the side. Look toward your right shoulder and, with every exhalation, stretch your right arm out a little more. If your right arm is high off the floor, rest it on a cushion to help you release. Inhale as you come back to the center. Repeat to the right.

bring the legs down to the floor

arm out at 45 degrees to your body

15   Get ready for the Final Relaxation. Lie on the floor with your knees bent and feet flat. Place your hands under your head and lift your head to look down your center line (see inset). Gently lay your head back down on the floor. Bring your arms out a little way from your body with your palms facing upward. Stretch one leg out and then the other leg out along the floor.

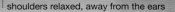

shoulders relaxed, away from the ears

16   Lie straight and relaxed, with a folded blanket under your head and something to cover you, if you like. Close your eyes. Now you are going to tense and relax each part of your body in turn.

>> **final relaxation**

17 Inhale and lift your right leg slightly off the floor. Tense the leg, exhale, and let it drop to the floor, relaxed. Repeat with your left leg.

lift one leg off
the floor

18 Inhale and lift your hips off the floor as you clench your buttocks together (see inset). Exhale and let them go. Inhale and lift your chest and back off the floor, bringing your shoulder blades together, and keeping your hips and head on the floor. Exhale and relax back down to the floor.

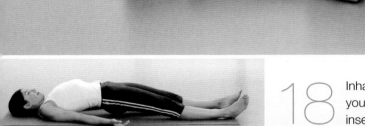

lift the chest off the floor

head remains
on the floor

hips remain
on the floor

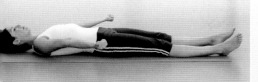

19 Inhale and lift both arms off the floor. Tense your arms, make fists (see inset), then stretch your fingers out. Exhale and let them drop back to the floor.

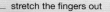

stretch the fingers out

20 Inhale and lift your shoulders, hunching them up tightly toward your ears. Exhale and let them drop, relaxed.

bring the shoulders up to the ears

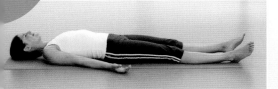

21 Inhale and screw your face up into a tiny ball toward your nose (see inset). Exhale and let go. Open your eyes wide and look backward. Open your mouth, stick your tongue out, and roar. Inhale and release.

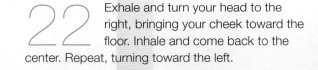

22 Exhale and turn your head to the right, bringing your cheek toward the floor. Inhale and come back to the center. Repeat, turning toward the left.

23 Feel comfortable and symmetrical. Close your eyes and systematically travel through every part of your body, from your toes to your forehead, relaxing every part as you go. Cover your eyes with an eye pad or folded cloth, if you like.

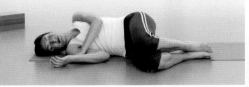

24 When you are ready to come up, roll onto the right side of your body (see inset). Stay here for a few seconds and then come up onto all fours to come up to kneeling. Bring your hands into prayer position, feeling calm and contented, and give thanks.

index

resources

General Fitness Resources

The American College of Sports Medicine
www.acsm.org
ACSM promotes and integrates scientific research, education, and practical applications of sports medicine and exercise science to maintain and enhance physical performance, fitness, health, and quality of life.

The American Council on Exercise
www.acefitness.org
ACE is a nonprofit organization committed to enriching quality of life through safe and effective physical activity. ACE protects society against ineffective fitness products, programs, and trends through its ongoing public education, outreach, and research. ACE sets certification and continuing education standards for fitness professionals.

The American Physical Therapy Association
www.APTA.org
The mission of the American Physical Therapy Association (APTA), the principal membership organization representing and promoting the profession of physical therapy, is to further the profession's role in the prevention, diagnosis, and treatment of movement dysfunctions and the enhancement of the physical health and functional abilities of members of the public.

IDEA
www.ideafit.com
IDEA is a worldwide membership organization providing health and fitness professionals with pertinent information, educational opportunities, career development, and industry leadership.

Yoga Alliance
www.yogaalliance.org
tel: 877-964-2255
Find a Yoga Alliance certified teacher or yoga center through this national Yoga Teacher's Registry.

Pilates Method Alliance
www.pilatesmethodalliance.org
PMA is an international organization that seeks to keep the Pilates Method pure. It is the gold-standard in the certification of the Pilates Method, and is a great resource for finding studios and teachers in your location.

Fitness Equipment

Hugger Mugger Yoga Products
www.huggermugger.com
tel: 800-473-4888
Stable, non-slip mats and clothing available for wholesale or retail.

Lululemon
www.lululemon.com
Functional and fashionable apparel for Pilates.

Manduka
www.manduka.com
tel: 805-544-3744
High-performance, ecologically friendly mats, bags, towels, accessories, and apparel.

Marika
www.marika.com
The softest fabrics and clever designs keep the Marika crowd completely loyal to the brand.

Topaz Medical
www.topazusa.com
e-mail: info@topazusa.com
tel: 800-264-5623
Specializes in rehabilitation exercise equipment, selling high-quality gel-filled medicine balls.

Yoga Retreats

Himalyan Institute
www.himalayaninstitute.org
tel: 800-822-4547
Headquartered in rural Pennsylvania, the center offers programs in hatha yoga, meditation, stress reduction, Ayurveda, nutrition, spirituality, and Eastern philosophy.

Kripalu Center for Yoga and Health
www.kripalu.org
tel: 866-200-5203
Retreat center in New England with everything from great yoga classes to massages. Kripalu hosts famous teachers in yoga, Buddhism, and other contemplative arts.